Dedication

I dedicate this book to my dear mother Shantabai and my dear father Dnyaneshwar, both since deceased. They loved me dearly and always kept my hands filled with their blessings.

Humbly theirs
Shantakumar Bhandarkar

HISTORY TAKING

Physical Examination for Medical Students and Students of Medicine

(Listen First, Listen Second)

by Dr. S.D. Bhandarkar, M.D., F.R.C.P.
Retired Honorary Professor and Head
Department of Endocrinology
Seth G.S. Medical College and K.E.M. Hospital, Mumbai
Co-author of Pharmacology and Pharmacotherapeutics

Dr. Mrs. Pallavi D. Bhandarkar M.S. (E.N.T.),
F.C.P.S., D.O.R.L., Dip. N.B., D.L.O. (London)
Consultant E.N.T. Surgeon, B.A.R.C. Hospital, Mumbai

Mrs. Archana P. Bhandarkar
B.Sc. (Nutrition), P.G. Dip. (Dietetics)
Nutritionist, Mumbai

Popular Prakashan
www.popularprakashan.com

Published by
Harsha Bhatkal for
POPULAR PRAKASHAN PVT. LTD.
301, Mahalaxmi Chambers
22, Bhulabhai Desai Road
Mumbai 400 026

First Published 2017

(4453)
ISBN: 978-81-7991-894-4

Design: Anjali Sawant

PRINTED IN INDIA
by Rama Printer
4743/23, Ansari Road, Darya Ganj
New Delhi-110002

Contents

Preface vii
Patient's Identifying Information xi
Equipment xiii

1. Timeline Table 1
2. Medical Record 5
3. What is Normal in Clinical Medicine? 7
4. Normal Physical Findings in Healthy Adults 10
5. Normal Ageing 25
6. Pregnant Women 30
7. Pillars of Clinical Medicine 32
8. Importance of Clinical Medicine 41
9. History Taking, Introduction 46
10. Present Illness 52
11. Diet and Physiological Functions 58
12. Specific Interrogation, Empathy, Associated Symptoms and Symptom Analysis 62
13. System Symptom Review (S.S.R.) 66
14. Past History 74
15. Personal and Social History 76
16. Family History 80
17. Allergy and Travel History 82
18. Physical Examination (P.E.), Introduction 84
19. Physical Examination, Principles 87

20. Valuation of Physical Signs 95
21. Measurement in Medicine 101
22. General Examination, Introduction 103
23. General Examination, Continued 107
24. Head and Neck 111
25. Skin, Breasts, Axillae and Upper Limbs 118
26. Thorax and Lungs 124
27. Cardiovascular and Lymphatic Systems 131
28. Abdomen 141
29. Groins, External Genitals and Lower Limbs 150
30. Physical Signs in Diabetes Mellitus 154
31. Central Nervous System 157
32. Diagnosis and Record Keeping 165

Appendices 170
List of Sources of Information Used 172

Preface

He who studies medicine without books sails an uncharted sea. He who studies medicine without seeing patients does not go to sea at all (Sir William Osler).

After finishing the pre-clinical courses, the **medical students** join the wards. In the first term, they are taught, in small batches, History Taking and Physical Examination of the patient **(bedside or clinical medicine)**. These are new subjects in which they must become skilled. They are also allotted patients to practice the new skills they are learning. They are confused about where to start and how to proceed. This book shows them the way to do it: how to take a good history and how to carry out a thorough physical examination. The students should record the history and the physical signs of the patients allotted to them, and get the record checked by the teacher. Because of the abundant new material added, this book will be helpful to **Medical students as well as to (Lifelong) Students of Medicine at all levels.**

Teaching theoretical aspects of medicine is beyond the scope of this book. For that purpose, the students have to purchase and read an appropriate textbook of medicine. The basic principles of clinical medicine remain the same whether you are learning/ practicing medicine, surgery or any subspeciality.

'History Taking' and 'What is Normal in Clinical Medicine?' are the most important topics in this book. This is not to say that physical examination is less important.

This book is about adults affected with problems in internal medicine and its subspecialities. It only touches upon problems in other specialities such as surgery, pediatrics, gynecology, orthopedics, ophthalmology and otorhinolaryngology.

The patient is referred to in the book as 'he' and not as 'he/she' or 'they' except in specific situations involving female patients.

This is the revised third edition of the book. In addition to revising the core text of the 2nd edition, I have added new topics to it in order to broaden the students' perspective of the scope and power of clinical medicine. The new topics are:

- Timeline of Important Events in The Development of Clinical Medicine.
- Medical Record.
- What is Normal in Medicine?
- The Pillars of Bedside (Clinical) Medicine.
- The Importance of History Taking and Physical Examination.
- Valuation of the Physical Signs.
- Measurement in Medicine.

The purpose of this book is:

- To stress the importance of history taking and physical examination upon the students.
- To teach them what questions to ask the patient and what physical examination to carry out. It is recommended that this book be carried on person to the ward and the O. P. D, and referred to frequently.
- To tell them in simple language some new ways of looking at Clinical Medicine such as 'What is Normal in Clinical Medicine?' and 'Valuation of Physical Signs'.

I hope the book fulfils that purpose.

I thank my colleague and friends Dr. Shreerang Godbole, Endocrinologist; Dr. Vishwas Mundale Ph.D.-Tech., Chemical Engineer; Dr. Sunil Pandya, Neurosurgeon; Dr. V.R. Mehta, Dermatologist; Dr. Mrs. Ashwini Bhalerao-Gandhi, Gynecologist; Dr. L.N. Vora, Orthopedic Surgeon; Dr. Rajeev Satoskar, Professor of Surgery, Dr. C.K. Ponde, Cardiologist for their helpful suggestions during this revision. Talking to Dr. Mundale on the telephone was 'distance education' on extra-medical topics to me.

My sincere thanks also to M/S.S.R. Systems (Total Solution for your Computer System) Andheri, Mumbai.

I also thank Mr. Harsha Bhatkal, our publisher, and the staff of Popular Prakashan Pvt. Ltd. for producing this book.

I especially thank my wife Kirtilata for making our house a home. Without her patience and indulgence, writing this book might not have been possible. Appreciation, suggestions and constructive criticism are welcome. They may please be sent to the publisher.

S.D. Bhandarkar

Patient's Identifying Information

Work is temple, and the patients are gods (Anonymous).

Record the following information carefully as this is also a document of medico-legal importance:

Patient's full name.

Patient's address in detail and telephone number.

Referred by Dr. ________________________________

Referring doctor's telephone number.

Date, time and place of examination.

Patient's nationality.

Age.:_______ Gender: (Male/Female/Other).

Marital status: Married/Single/Widowed/Divorced.

Educational status.

Occupation.

Write in bold letters such information as (1) Allergy or intolerance to any drug or food; (2) Patient being treated currently with a corticosteroid, an oral anticoagulant or aspirin in men and women; and an oral contraceptive in women.

Equipment

The students and the practicing clinicians should carry the following equipment with them to the ward:

- A stethoscope.
- A pen torch.
- A ruler.
- A soft but non-stretchable measuring tape.
- A tendon hammer.
- Two tuning forks: 128 cps and 256 cps.
- A magnifying lens.
- A small box containing cotton, pins and pieces of colored cloth or paper.
- An ophthalmoscope.
- A standardized nylon hair (monofilament) to test sensation on the sole in diabetic patients.
- A simple otoscope.

Chapter 1

Timeline Table

Hippocrates established medicine as a respectable, independent profession. He described many physical signs, Hippocratic facies being one.

Osler established and popularized Clinical Medicine in the US. During his lifetime and thereafter, his method of bedside (clinical) medicine spread all over the US and the world. But, after the 1940s, clinical medicine waned in popularity, especially in the US because of:

(a) The development of super-technologies: ultrsonography, C.T. scan, M.R.I. scan and advanced laboratory technology.

(b) The replacement of traditional, bedside (clinical) teaching by computer-assisted teaching in a ward side-room; and (c) Computerized, multiple-choice, question papers in the board examinations. The National Board of Medical Examiners (N.B.E.M.) in the US has declared that the traditional clinical assessment (long case, short case and viva) in the old one-to-one style for large numbers of aspirants is very expensive and not practicable.

"The decline of clinical medicine is also due to the over-lecturing, and under-teaching of clinical medicine" (J. Willis Hurst).

Arnold Relman (1923-2014), a medical scholar and a long-time chief editor of N.E.J.M., passed away in 2014. He gave a patient's eye view of his own ordeal and subsequent recovery from a neck injury. He said "new technologies and electronic record keeping affect how doctors do their work. Attention to the masses of data generated by laboratory and imaging studies has shifted their focus away from the patient. Doctors now spend more time with their computers than at the bedside; whatever personal care patients now get is mostly from the nurses".

Professor Abraham Verghese, at the Stanford University School of Medicine, has made it his life's mission to restore clinical medicine to its Oslerian glory; but see the N.E.B. M.'s declaration above. Money matters. How you spend it is your choice.

Patient history: Paying attention to the patient's history has been practiced since ancient times. The Chinese physicians as well as Sushrut, Charak and Hippocrates were especially skilled in that art. Around AD 1700, the Dutch physician Hermann Boerhaave laid the foundation of bedside medicine with the aid of detailed history and limited physical examination. Percussion was yet to be discovered and auscultation was yet to be invented.

The model of modern, structured history of the patient was developed by the French school of medicine, especially Louis, Corvisart and others. Willium Osler used to lay great stress upon History Taking. He used to say "Listen to the patient; he is telling you the diagnosis". Further, he wished that the following epitaph be inscribed on his tombstone. "He used to take a small number of students to the ward, and teach them medicine". The art of history taking further expanded as the number of medical specialties grew in the twentieth century. But, in the second half of the twentieth century, clinical medicine met with a rough spot by having to compete with computer-assisted medical history and records, for the reasons detailed above. The tussle still goes on.

Timeline of Clinical Medicine

Period/ Year	Era/Place of work	Physician	Major contribution
5000-6000 BC	Ancient Indian medicine	Collective work	Rugved, which contains references to medicine
c 5000 BC	Traditional Chinese medicine	Zhang Zhonjing	History and elementary physical examination
c 3300 BC	Ancient Egyptian medicine	Imhotep	Polymath, including medicine. Edwyn Smith Papyrus
600 BC	Traditional Indian (Ayurvedic) medicine	Sushrut	Versatile surgeon. Sushrut Samhita
c 400 BC	Greek med-icine	*Hippocrates	Refined history taking and physical examination
100 BC	Traditional Indian (Ayurvedic) medicine	Charak	History and elementary physical examination. Charak Samhita
c AD 130-201	Greek medicine	Claudius Galen	Talented physician
AD 1543	What is currently Belgium	Andrea Vesalius	Founder of human anatomy
AD 1666	UK	Thomas Sydenham	Taught medicine in the ward. Known as the English Hyppocrates
c 1700	Holland	Hermann Boerhaave	Founder of bedside medicine

AD 1761	Austria	Leopold Auenbruggeer	Discovered clinical percussion
AD 1761	Italy	Giovanni Morgagni	Founder of pathological anatomy
AD 1816	France	Rene Laennec	Invented stethoscope
AD 1800-1850	France	Pierre Louis and others	Developed French School of medicine
AD 1850	Germany	Hermann Helmholtz	Invented direct vision ophthalmoscope
AD 1871	Germany	Carl Wunderlich	Invented clinical thermometer
AD 1875	Germany	Erb and Westphal	Invented reflex hammer
AD 1830-1900	Germany	Johaness Muller	Developed German School of medicine
AD 1890s	Johns Hopkins in U.S.A.; then Oxford in U.K.	Sir William Osler	Established clinical methods in medicine
AD 1896	Italy	Riva-Rocci	Invented sphygmomanometer
AD 2007 to date	Stanford University School of Medicine in U.S.A.	Abraham Verghese	Mission to re-vitalize clinical medicine

Chapter 2

Medical Record

Discharge status: Alive, without permission (from an actual medical record as dictated by a physician).

(Source: The Internet)
(Also see Chapters 19 and 32.)

The medical record comprises the systematic documentation of a single patient's medical history and his care now and across all future time. It includes 'notes' **written** by the consultant and the residents, recording: (a) History, (b) Findings of physical examination, (c) Laboratory and imaging test results, (d) Diagnosis and the reasons for it, (e) Treatment administered and response to it (including complications), (f) Prescription for further treatment and (g) Follow up notes, all stored in an easily accessible folder. Such a record may also be **digital**.

The medical record is confidential, and should be accessible immediately only to authorized persons, when required. It may be transferred to another physician with the written permission of the patient or his care giver, if the patient is not in a condition to make that decision. The patient has the right to read his own medical record, and to obtain certified copies of it. Further, it has to be produced in a court-of–law upon judge's order.

A medical record serves multiple purposes: As a patient-service record, as an academic record and as a medico-legal record. Therefore, a good medical record should conform to the following norms:

- If it is hand-written, it should be tidy, legible and to the point; neither verbose nor terse, and unambiguous. It may also be digital.

- There should be **no use of abbreviation of phrases and words** in the medical record e.g. EOF for edema of feet; 'u' for you or for unit; IU for international unit; r for are (internet SMS language). Other examples of unacceptable abbreviations are: OD for daily; QOD for every other day; MS for morphine sulfate or magnesium sulfate. These abbreviations are **prohibited** by Ninth Joint Commission, U.S., (2009). They may be misread, or one mistaken for another, with disastrous result.
- It should be rapidly accessible to authorized persons at all times. In 1960-1961, in the Medical Records Department of The Western Infirmary in Glasgow, U.K., a notice board said, "The difficult, we do immediately; the impossible takes time". The free availability and use of computers in the medical establishments have made the instant access to stored data a reality.

Chapter 3

What is Normal in Clinical Medicine?

It seems to me to be fundamental that doctors should be thoroughly conversant with the normal, normal variations and the reasons for those variations. They need this as a basis for the diagnosis of the abnormal (1981; R.S. Illingworth, Professor of Pediatrics).

This question is difficult to answer because there is no universally agreed upon definition of normal. The word is used by different workers in different senses in different contexts.

There is not one, absolute, normal value for an **appearance**, a measurable **object**, or an **attribute**. An attribute is a characteristic, inherent quality of an object, generally good, a part of the human body in this case. An appearance, an object, an attribute and a number can be given a **name** (e.g. a book, an egg which are nouns); or (black, white, clear, beautiful; or five, seven which are adjectives). **The normal is** the average (the mean or the median) **of a set of values, between two values (a range) found in a sample of the population.** Most biological objects and attributes are liable to vary. In clinical medicine, we deal with anatomical variation i.e. variation in the form, shape and size (a number) of human body or its parts.

A **variable** is something which is liable to vary qualitatively or quantitatively. The values within a given set are **variants** of each other. A variant which is close to the average of a set (after the outliers are excluded) is called a **normal variant**. The literature on biology gives many such expected ranges.

Clinicians generally label as clinically normal, a person: Who has no complaints and no abnormality on physical examination, and is, therefore, healthy according to the W.H.O. definition which is "health is a state of complete physical, mental and social well being, and not merely absence of disease or infirmity".

and

He has the value of a physical attribute, perceived by human senses or by measurement, which

(1) Is not grossly different from that of the average of the same category.

(2) Permits normal functioning of the part or the organ affected.

(3) Is not causing ill health.

(4) Does not (by collective knowledge) predict a possible future illness. Such a piece of knowledge is called **a risk factor.**

(5) Is not known to affect longevity adversely; and

(6) Does not require medical intervention at the material time.

Some common examples of normal variants are: stature; body hair distribution and age at commencement and completion of sexual maturity. Such variations are genetic in origin. One must be careful in labeling them as abnormal.

If you subject a person to one of the modern 'Gold Standard' tests such as ultrasonography, C.T. scan or M.R.I. scan, it may show a small difference in the shape, size or functioning from that in most other persons in the same category. If the person with such a small difference satisfies the above mentioned criteria, he can be said to be a **normal variant**; he should be reassured that he is normal, and is best left alone.

The following are some more examples of normal variants seen **in adults**. They are shown here to sensitize the students of medicine to possibility of their occurrence.

- Medullated nerve fibres in the optic fundi.
- Slightly R or L deviated uvula or penis.
- A few hair on the areolae of the breast of some healthy women.
- A few coarse hair on the chin in postmenopausal women.
- Impalpable ulnar artery pulse.
- Palpable lymph nodes (except trochlear, infraclavicular and supraclavicular) smaller than 1 cm in diameter.
- Barrel chest (round thoracic cage) in the absence of emphysema.
- Idiopathic galactorrhoea (a diagnosis by exclusion).
- B.P. 140-150/70-80 in those 80 years and older (Bates).
- Bilaterally diminished or absent tendon reflexes, especially in the elderly.
- A few beats of nystagmus on extreme lateral gaze if the pupillary reactions are normal.
- In lighter-skinned people, the gums are pale or coral pink and lightly stippled. In darker-skinned people, they may be diffusely or partly brown.

For more examples of normal variants, see chapters on Physical Examination. The message, therefore, is "In clinical work, keep the normal variant in mind".

Chapter 4

Normal Physical Findings in Healthy Adults

Data on 'What is Clinically Normal' is scarce because the funding agencies are reluctant to sanction funds for simple research projects. "Normal need not apply", they seem to imply (Thomas Goetz, the Deputy Editor of Wired Magazine, Issue 16.05).

Normal Physical Findings are found on **observation** (visual inspection plus minimal palpation as required) of different parts of the body in healthy adults. Order of body parts in the second table below is roughly 'head to toe'.

Repeated examination of **normal** persons helps you to recognize the **abnormal** features in **patients**. The following tables describe the normal physical findings (I do not call them *physical signs* in normal people) on observation. The skin is the largest organ in the body (16% of the body weight, and 1.2 to 2.3 square metres in area). It is easily accessible to observation; therefore it is a good mirror to health.

There are two paragraphs on normal physical findings below, which list the entries in the table in two ways. If you want to look up, say, how the normal thorax looks like and feels, read the alphabetical list first. If it is there in that list, go to the head-toe paragraph to locate and read it. I am aware that the table is incomplete. An attempt will be made to correct this shortcoming in the next edition.

Alphabetical list

Abdomen; Antecubital fossa and elbow; Axillae; Body structure; Breasts; Chest, back; Chest, front and sides; Ears;

External genitals; Eyes; Face; Feet; Forearms; Gait; General appearance; Groins; Hair colours; Hands; Head; Height; Knees; Legs; Lips; Lower jaw; Lymph nodes; Mons pubis; Mouth; Neck, front; Nose; Salivary glands; Scalp hair; Shoulders and hips; Skin; Thighs; Throat; Upper arms; US/LS ratio; Voice.

Head-to-toe list

General appearance; Voice; Height; Body structure; Skin; Head; Scalp hair; Hair colours; Face; Lower jaw; Salivary glands; Lips; Mouth; Nose; Throat; Ears, Eyes; Lymph nodes; Neck, front; Breasts; Chest, front and sides; Shoulders and hips; Axillae; Upper arms; Antecubital fossae and elbows; Forearms; Hands; Chest, back; Abdomen; Mons pubis; External genitals; Groins; Thighs; Knees; Legs; Feet; US/LS ratio; Gait.

A large amount of information can be gathered by the trained eye and limited use of hands (= observation). To facilitate your learning, we give below the normal appearances and feel of many of the parts in the adult male and female bodies from head to toe. The term 'Normal variant' and its importance are explained in Chapter 3.

Part of the body	**Men**	**Women Examine in the presence of another lady**
General appearance	Tough = masculine. May be indifferently groomed and/or untidily dressed. Such a man may be lazy or a rebel against the establishment.	Delicate = feminine. Carefully groomed and tidily dressed, appropriately for age. A woman who is not so may be either ill or unhappy.
Voice	Low pitched.	High pitched.
Height	All-India average 165 cm.	All-India average 152 cm.

Body structure	Heavier.	Ligher.
Skin: Normal skin varies a lot in different parts of the body. So it is difficult to give a unified description of it. The skin of other parts of the body than the face should be examined along with the regional examination of the part concerned.	Less soft and less smooth. Thicker. Darker. Less hydrated. Oily in youth. May become dry and rough especially with ageing. The skin of the armpits, groins and genitals is darker than the skin over the rest of the body. **Cellulite:** 10% of patients with cellulite are obese men. Commoner in older than in younger persons. **Terminai hair:** Long or short, straight and soft or curly and wiry; variably dense, on the scalp, face (moustache and beard), eyelashes, eyebrows, trunk, upper arms, forearms, thighs, legs, axillae and mons pubis in men. Few men wear the protective sun screen. Therefore, more prone than women to develop acne and skin cancer. Palms and soles are hairless.	Softer and smoother. Less oily. Better hydrated. Lighter coloured. Thinner and therefore, facial wrinkling affects ageing women more than ageing men. UV exposure in sunshine (natural) and indoors (artificial) may tan it. But more women than men use cosmetics and protective sun screen. **Vellus hair:** Short, fine, light coloured and barely noticeable; cover face, trunk, upper arms and thighs in women. **Terminal hair:** Outer ⅔rds of the external auditory canal has terminal hair in both genders. Terminal hair are present on the scalp, in eyelashes, eyebrows, forearms, legs, axillae and on mons pubis in women. The upper pubic hair line is horizontal. **Cellulite on thighs and buttocks:** 90% of the patients with cellulite are obese women. Starting at youth, it frequency increases with age.

Head	Larger. About 56 cm in circumference. Varies in shape but symmetrical. Lumpy in the elderly.	Smaller. The rest is same.
Scalp hair	Are terminal hair (see above). Graying and baldness increase with age. Density variable. Worn short. Bitemporal recession of frontal hair line present in adults.	Are terminal hair. Worn long or short. Well groomed and oiled and therefore lustrous. No temporal recession. Frontal hair line horizontal. The rest is same.
Hair colours	The **natural colours** of terminal hair are black, brown, blond, red and white. White hair are due to absence of melanin. Other colours are due to varying amounts and proportions of eumelanin and pheomelanin in a given hair. Grey appearance is due to less melanin than normal, on its way to becoming white.	Some men and women like to alter the hair colour with synthetic chemicals. The rest same.
Face	Symmetrical, mobile and expressive. May be plump. Dry to oily. Complexion variable. Variable quantity of black terminal hair: beard, moustache, eyelashes and eyebrows. The rest of the face vellus hair.	Vellus hair only, except eyebrows and eyelids. No beard or moustache. Less prone to acne. Chloasma during and lifelong after pregnancy. The rest is same.
Lower jaw	Symmetrical but shape may be variable.	Same.

Salivary glands	Normal parotid and submandibular glands are not palpable. The openings of their ducts may be seen in the mouth.	Same.
Lips	Less pink. Less full. Shrink with age and with excessive exposure to sunshine.	Pinker. Fuller. Lipstick may protect against sunshine, but the chemicals contained in it may cause damage. Shrink with age.
Mouth	Not open during quiet breathing. Teeth variably clean, white, and aligned. Gums pink and healthy. Tongue symmetrical, moist, pink; dorsal surface rough because of taste buds. Oral mucosa may have dark patches in certain races. No foul smell.	Same.
Nose	Larger and of variable shape. No running of nose Alae nasi not moving during quiet breathing. Dust filtering terminal hair present.	Smaller. The rest is same.
Throat	Mucosa pink; smooth/ or granular. Tonsils vary in size from barely visible to large. *Large* tonsils are not *necessarily* abnormal. Uvula central; a slight deviation to right or left is a *normal variant*.	Same.

Eyes	Bilaterally symmetrical. Palpebral fissure horizontal or sloping slightly downwards from medial to lateral. Sloping upwards from medial to lateral in people of Mongolian origin. Cornea transparent. Iris variably coloured, black, grey, brown, blue or green. Blinking 10-20/minute. White of the eye (sclera) not visible either above or below the cornea; upper ⅓rd of cornea is covered by upper eyelid. Fine bulbar conjunctival and sub-conjunctival blood vessels seen. Sclera is avascular. It may be brownish muddy in the inter-palpabral fissure; differentiate from jaundice. Conjunctiva healthy pink. Eyeballs not protruding; but mild proptosis may be familial (*a normal variant*). Moving in all directions with their long axes parallel. Eversion of lower eyelids with watering in the old. Arcus senilis may be seen in the elderly.	Same.

Ears: auricles (pinnae) and external auditory canal	Shape and size variable. Not low set (see Chapter 24 for definition). Long terminal hair may be present on the pinna, especially in the elderly. Outer ⅔rds of the external auditory canal is of cartilage, covered by skin, containing wax-secreting glands and terminal hair in both genders. The inner ⅓ rd is of bone, without skin covering it. Tympanic membrane concave on otoscopy.	No terminal hair on the pinna. Like in men, terminal hair present on the outer two thirds of external auditory canal. The rest is same.
Neck, front	The neck is shorter and stouter. Thyroid cartilage (Adam's apple) is prominent and moves up and down during swallowing. Carotid pulsation is seen and felt, but venous pulsation is only seen. Aortic pulsation may be visible in suprasternal notch. Thyroid gland may be just visible (goiter) with tangential light; less often than in women. Trachea central. Tiny, shotty lymph nodes may be felt in the posterior triangles.	The neck is slender and longer. Thyroid cartilage less prominent than in men. A just visible thyroid (goiter) more frequent than in men; it enlarges further slightly during pregnancy. The rest is same.
Shoulders and hips	Shoulders broader than hips. All movements free.	Hips broader than shoulders; and waist (W/H ratio < 1.00)

Lymph nodes	They are present in groups at many sites in the body. Only superficial i.e. subcutaneous lymph nodes are clinically palpable. They vary in size from barely palpable to 1cm in diameter, without a focus of disease. They are discrete, non-adherent, not caseous (meaning not softened by central necrosis, not tender), not hard. They are movable from side to side and up-and-down on physical examination with the patient vertical. Arterioles and bits of muscles which mimic lymph nodes are not movable in this manner. Further, the artery pulsates; a lymph node does not. Lymph nodes diminish in size with age; any easily palpable lymph nodes in the elderly are worrisome. Many other conditions may mimic a lymph node (see Mosby's book for a complete list).	Same as in men, except those related to genitals and breasts.
Axillae	Terminal hair, variable in density. Scantier in old age. Dark skin pigmentation +/-. Smelly in adults.	Palpable axillary tail of the breast may mimic a lump in the axilla. The rest is same.

Breasts	Nipples and areolae, and perhaps a supernumerary nipple seen. Gynecomastia (enlarged breast in a male) seen during normal puberty, in old men and those on certain drugs.	Breasts, nipples and areolae seen prominently. Skin is smooth. In most women, both nipples are everted; but one nipple or both may be flat or inverted in a few. Nipples and areolae are pigmented brown to black; they become darker during pregnancy. No nipple discharge except during pregnancy, lactation and while on certain drugs. Supernumerary nipples may be present. Breasts vary very much in size and shape from woman to woman. The two breasts may differ in size. Round or conical, and full in the young; flattened and sagging in the elderly. In the young female, most of a breast feels soft due to fat both in front and behind it, with interspersed firm areas due to glandular tissue; it may feel granular if palpated between tips of two fingers. In the elderly, it feels soft due to shrinking of glandular tissue. **But, there is no lump palpable to the 'flat of the hand'** (see Chapter 19).

		A palpable part extends into the axilla (tail of the breast). Breasts may be tender during mammary growth during puberty; pre-menstrually; during pregnancy; and during combined oral contraceptive therapy.
Upper arms	Muscular and strong. The dominant arm is more muscular. Terminal hair may be present.	Less muscular and less strong. Only vellus hair are present.
Forearms	More muscular and stronger; prominent veins may be seen. Terminal hair are commonly present.	Less muscular and less strong. The veins are covered by fat and hidden. Terminal hair may be present.
Antecubital fossa and elbow	Prominent antecubital vein seen. Carrying angle (Normal range 5-15 degrees), smaller than in women.	Veins less prominent. Carrying angle (Normal range 5-15 degrees), larger than in men.
Mons pubis	Covered by terminal hair. Has a pad of fat underneath the skin. Upper hairline may rise in the midline up the linea alba.	Also called mons veneris in the female. Covered by terminal hair. Has a pad of fat underneath the skin Upper hairline is horizontal.
Groins	No lump nor impulse on coughing. A few lymph nodes may be palpable.	Same.

Hands	Larger but less flexible and less dexterous. The handgrip is stronger (Power grip). Ten per cent of all people are left handed; percentage frequency is higher in men than in women. Joints are supple and move freely through the entire range. Veins are more prominent on the dorsum of the hands. Nails flat in long axis, convex in short axis. The linear axes of the forearm and the hand are in the same line. Palms soft or rough (Normal variants.) In addition, they may be rough because of manual labour.	Smaller but more flexible and more dexterous. The handgrip is less strong but hands have more finesse at handling small, delicate objects such as threading a needle and assembling electronic components (Precision grip). Veins less prominent than in men. Fewer women than men are left-handed. The rest is same.
Abdomen	Flat to bulging. No tenderness. Waist is the narrowest part of the trunk. Excess fat is deposited on waist in obesity. (Apple shaped). Well toned abdominal muscles may be seen in heavy exercisers. Covered variably by terminal hair. Umbilicus moderately deep. No mass seen. No veins visible. Aortic pulsation may be seen in thin persons. No impulse on coughing. No intestinal coils visible.	Excess fat may be deposited on hips, buttocks and thighs in obesity. (Pear shaped). Supra-pubic region may be slightly bulging. Abdomen progressively more bulging in pregnancy. Skin covered by vellus hair. The rest is same.

Chest, back	Two sides symmetrical and move equally during breathing. Cervical lordosis, dorsal kyphosis and lumbar lordosis can be appreciated. Spinous process of seventh cervical vertebra prominent; it is an anatomical landmark.	Same.
Chest, front and sides	Sterno-manubrial junction prominent and is an anatomical landmark. Chest variably covered with terminal hair. Pale striae of obesity may be seen. Ribs with intercostal spaces seen. No intercostal or suprasternal retraction during breathing. Chest wall seen moving equally on both sides with breathing. Thoracic breathing more prominently visible while sitting. Diaphragmatic breathing more prominently visible while supine (Bates). Normal apical cardiac impulse seen in left fifth interspace in thin men. Precordium not moving.	Apical cardiac impulse is difficult to find because of being covered by left breast. Chest covered by vellus hair except a terminal hair or two on the areolae. The rest are same.
Feet	Larger. Slight edema of the feet and ankles may be present by the evening in the elderly. Arches normal.	Smaller. Edema of the feet in normal pregnancy. The rest same.

External genitals	They are (1) **Mons pubis** (2) **Penis** (flaccid, normal length 3-4"; erect, 5½ -6"); may deviate a little to R or L. (3) **Scrotum**: no scrotal swelling seen (4) **Testes** 10-20 ml (by orchidometry); (5) One testis, more commonly left, hangs lower than the right. This probably prevents the trauma they would incur by knocking against each other, were they hanging at the same level (6) Testes are very sensitive; they hurt even on slight pressure.	All the external genitals considered together are called the **vulva**. They are (1) **Mons pubis**. (2) Left and right. **Labia majora**. They are plump (due to a subcutaneous pad of fat) and hairy. The two meet in the midline to form the **pudendal cleft.** (3) **Left and right labia minora** are wihin the labia majora. They have no pad of fat and are thin; they are also hairless. They line the labia majora from within. (4) Labia majora and labia minora cover and protect all other external genitalia viz. the **clitoris, urethral orifice, vaginal introitus and hymen.** (5) The labia minora vary in length and width, and may or may not protrude dimensions are largely responsible for the variety of appearances of the vulva (normal variants). (6) **Clitoris**, the female equivalent of the male penis, is an erectile organ. Normally, it measures up to 1.0 cm in length and up to 0.7 cm in breadth

		at the base. **Clitoral index** (length mm x breadth mm), if higher than 35.00, indicates clitoromegaly and, hyper-androgenism needs to be ruled out (William's Endocrinology)
Knees	Five degrees valgus. Movements full and free.	Same.
Legs	Prominent gastrocnemius in gymnasts. Terminal hair present.	Less muscular than in men. Terminal hair may be present.
Upper segment (US)/Lower segment (LS) ratio	US / LS ratio 1.00: 1.00	US/LS ratio 1.00/1.00 In some healthy women, some of them models or athletes, the legs are very long, and the ratio may be down to 1.00/1.40 (0.70). Such long legs are considered a sign of beauty. This is not hypogonadism unless the arm span also exceeds the total height by more than 5.00 cm.
Gait	**Heel-toe gait** (see following page) Arms swinging by the side.	Same.
Thighs	Like upper arms. Variably hairy (terminal hair). Cellulite: see above	Covered by velllus hair. Commonly plump. Cellulite: see above.

While walking, one heel is lifted from the floor, followed by lifting of the toes. This is followed by the heel touching the ground first and then the toes. The other foot follows suit. This is the normal 'heel-toe' gait and is common to the male and the female.

(For further discussion on average Indian height, see Chapter 23.)

Chapter 5

Normal Ageing

In the end, it's not the years in your life that matters. It is the life in your years (Abraham Lincoln).

There is no universally agreed upon definition of the term 'elderly'. In their paper titled 'Definition of an older or elderly person' the WHO states as follows "Most developed world countries have accepted the chronological age of 65 years as a definition of 'an elderly or older' person..." However, the WHO does not give its own definition. Nevertheless, 65 years or older is considered as the international definition of older adults i.e. the elderly. In India, the dividing line between middle age and old age (Senior Citizens) is 60 years at present.

A human being starts ageing the day he is born. He first grows up in height till the end of puberty, and then matures physically and mentally to a peak until age 25-30 years. Most organs start declining in function slowly (1-2 per cent a year) but irreversibly, at around 30 years of age. Some organs may begin this process even earlier. This decline can be demonstrated quantitatively and convincingly by serial measurements of Bone Mineral Density (B.M.D.) which declines with age; and serum creatinine which rises with age, from about thirty years of age. The other organs follow suit. The adults age at different rates.

In healthy persons, this decline is a continuous process which cannot be halted nor reversed. But, the progress of its clinical manifestations can be slowed by a healthy life style (proper nutrition, regular physical activity, periodic medical check up, recommended immunizations and medications, and avoidance of known 'risk factors'. They are tobacco, alcohol and other recreational drugs:) (a) Legally permitted drugs such as psychotropic drugs; and (b) Drugs of abuse (also called street drugs)). Even with all these precautions, the body ages from wear and tear, unknown, undetected or ignored 'risk factors', unavoidable environmental toxins, infections and cancer, leave alone accidents.

When may we call a person old? For that purpose, the focus has shifted from the chronological age to the age at which the individual's ability to look after himself (activities of daily living, A.D.L.s) starts waning. Age for beginning of decline in ability to meet the A.D.Ls. is variable. In spite of this decline, most organ-functions remain adequate for good health for long periods of time.

There are some *fortunate* persons who do not appear to have been even touched by the internal and external risk factors such as metabolic disease, infections and environmental toxins, which are otherwise commonplace. They live a full active life till 100 years of age. We do not understand how this happens. Studies have shown that genes account for approximately 20 per cent of the probability of living till 100 years of age; healthy lifestyle accounts for another 20% to 30%. (Bates). That adds to about 50%; what accounts for the remaining 50% is a mystery. *Possibly good fortune.* And, it has recently been suggested that people who feel younger than their actual age and behave likewise (The Young at Heart) have lower mortality (J A M A).

In the elderly persons, it is important to differentiate between (a) Symptoms and signs of **primary ageing (senescence)** due to a natural decline in the organ functions, independently of any disease or trauma. This must be established by a detailed history, thorough physical examination and selective testing; and (b) Symptoms due to disease, including obesity and its consequences, under-nutrition, and manifestations of disease of one type or another (**secondary ageing**).

Primary ageing requires periodic monitoring and repeated reminders on continuing 'healthy living' (see above), and on promoting agreeable interrelationships within the family, which create in the beneficiary a feeling of being wanted and of being cared for. **Secondary ageing** requires investigation and advice about medical management and perhaps a care giver. In both groups, "The secret of the care of the patient is in caring for the patient" (Francis Peabody).

As each individual ages at his own unique rate, comparison with other people of the same age gives only limited information. A better comparison is with what that person was like in his own past, as judged by measurements (see above) or by detailed history and physical examination; the structure of history taking and physical examination needs to be modified from that used in younger persons. This may be difficult as the life expectation of the population continues to rise all the time. As it were, as each person continues to live beyond 30 years of age, he is a diminished and diminishing replica of himself in his younger days.

As constraints of space do not permit me to give the complete list of manifestation of primary ageing, I will give some examples of some symptoms in primary ageing.

(1) **General**: The ageing person tends to get tired more easily, and takes longer time to recover after rest or sleep. Restful night sleep becomes shorter. He is less tolerant of changes in ambient temperature e. g. he becomes cold intolerant. His appetite diminishes. He may become compulsive and his things must be found exactly at the same place. Life-long habits do not change easily and adaptation to new environment may be difficult. He may become touchy. Short term memoıy declines (benign forgetfulness), but the long term memory remains unchanged. Learning new skills may become difficult. Constipation is common. His hearing, especially for higher tones, diminishes.

He needs more light to read because of declining in dark-adaptation. He looks paler. His thirst diminishes and he is liable to develop dehydration more easily. He may have postural edema of feet and nocturia.

As against these negative points, he is likely to be more experienced, more knowledgeable and wiser. He may mellow out and become more loving and more accommodating, especially after grandchildren are born.

(2) **Specific**: Shortness of breath is common. Coughing is less effective in expelling the sputum. Cardiac murmurs are more ominous than in the young. Systolic blood pressure tends to rise. Skin becomes dry; and itching is common. Baldness of the skull may occur in both men and women. Women may develop a few coarse facial hair. Axillary, pubic, truncal and limb hair tend to diminish in both genders. Physically, he may become less strong and flabby; and stoops forward. His hands and even the head may shake. Gait may become slower. Hands may become less dexterous. Skeletal muscles atrophy (sarcopenia). Vibration sense and ankle reflexes diminish (Neurology of old age). Teeth tend to fall, and mouth tends to become dry. Frequency of palpable lymph nodes diminishes; and therefore palpable lymph nodes in an old man are worrisome. In women, breasts diminish in size, sag and feel softer but granular or even nodular. A hard, irregularly shaped lump in the breast, *palpable to the flat of the hand*, is an ominous finding (cancer). Accumulation of fat on the abdomen is common. Abdomen becomes softer and may be protruding. Sexual interest may remain the same, but performance decreases. Penis and testes become smaller. Extensive changes in external and internal genital organs occur in women due to estrogen loss at menopause. That may cause symptoms. Therefore, the women must be examined carefully so as not to miss a treatable condition. Menopausal hot flashes are common and may respond to reassurance or may need estrogen

replacement. Aching in body is common. Posture may be bent forward due to dorsal kyphoscoliosis, and height may diminish due to primary (or secondary) spinal osteoporosis.

In the elderly, the stress should be on establishing that the patient is ageing normally and has no disease. This is unlike in young adults where the stress is on finding a disease, and if one exists, treating it. That is clinical wisdom. Do not do sophisticated tests merely because it is possible to do them. Clinical acumen and clinical wisdom both should be cultivated as the physician's age and experience grow.

Activities of daily life (See Chapter 15).

Chapter 6

Pregnant Women

Feeling fat lasts nine months, but the joy of becoming a mom lasts for ever (attributed to Nikki Dalton).

Many physiologic changes occur in the female body during pregnancy, and may cause a variety of symptoms. Some of the symptoms, such as nausea, vomiting and backache are unpleasant. But, because the physiologic changes are mainly beneficial and even protective (enlarged blood volume protects against ill effects of bleeding during delivery), we may call the resulting symptoms normal, or at least acceptable.

The changes and symptoms are:

(1) Optimum weight gain.

(2) Early nausea and vomiting.

(3) Hyperpnoea which is thought of by the women as breathlessness.

(4) Gastroesophageal reflux and heartburn.

(5) Backache.

(6) Physiological anemia and edema of the feet; edema of the hands and the face is abnormal.

(7) Breasts enlarge and become more vascular, tender and nodular; nipple discharge and exaggerated venous pattern on the breasts are common. Nipples become darker, larger and more erectile; the areolae enlarge and become darker. Some women secrete colostrums in second and third trimesters.

(8) Increased vaginal discharge without foul smell, urinary frequency or vaginal itching may occur.

(9) Spider angiomas may be seen.

(10) Increased urinary frequency.

(11) Constipation is common.

(13) Just visible or palpable, diffuse goiter may be seen; and

(14) Melasma or chloasma, brownish dark cutaneous areas on the forehead, face and nose, tend to occur commonly.

Most of these changes disappear in course of time after the delivery; some such as chloasma are permanent.

Chapter 7

Pillars of Clinical Medicine

Describe first, without diagnosing (Mosby's book).

There are several ways of teaching and learning medicine. They are:

(1) **Bedside, also called clinical, method**: This method was initiated by Boerehaave in around AD 1700, but was widely popularized by William Osler in the U.S. more than a hundred years ago, and comprises **teaching a small batch of students in the presence of the patient (patient centered) in a medical college.** It consists of a three-way interaction among the patient, the students and the teacher. It is popularly known as 'Taking a Clinic'.

Its components are:

- The **presentation**, by the student-in-charge, of the patient's case history, and the abnormal physical signs he has found in the patient. This is followed by a free-for-all discussion on the presented material under the guidance of the teacher. The teacher appreciates the good points in the presentation, corrects the errors and encourages mutual questions and answers among all those present, about all aspects of the patient's illness. In addition, the teacher may give the students additional information such as the historical aspects of the patient's disease, an interesting anecdote about the same or about the discoverer of the disease or about its treatment, and so on. Examples are how penicillin and oral antidiabetic drugs were discovered.

There are no limits to the discussion as long as it is restricted to the illness of the patient under consideration.

- The teacher **demonstrates**, on the patient, and occasionally on a student, the correct way of eliciting physical signs such as examination for lymph nodes and spleen, pupillary signs, the ankle jerk and so on.
- In addition, by watching how the teacher talks to and behaves with the patient, the students learn **bedside manners**. *The students learn clinical medicine by imitating the teacher.* If they are fortunate, they may even find a role-model among their teachers.
- The patient's illness then comes alive in all its aspects and is remembered easily by the students. The essence of such interaction is a good patient history, the findings on a thorough physical examination, and discussion in the presence of the patient.

(2) **The non-clinical methods are:**

(a) Classroom lectures; (b) Tutorials; (c) Journal club; (d) Seminars; and (e) Home assignments.

These are carried out in the absence of the patient.

(3) **Computer-assisted methods**:

- The **desktop** method which implies: (a) Entering patient's history into the computer during the patient's interview itself; and (b) A discussion of history, physical signs, and laboratory and imaging results, all stored in a computer, in the side-room, but in the absence of the patient. The patient is seen only on admission and infrequently thereafter (Arnold Relman, personal experience, see Chapter 1). The fresh data are added to the computer at the physician's/resident's convenience or automatically, directly from the laboratory.

- This method gives the students the wrong message that discussing the stored data is more important than seeing the patient in person frequently, for follow-up. They do not see the nuances of a follow up examination to which the experienced clinicians attach so much importance. Another important disadvantage is that the computer cannot detect non-verbal communication (Chapter 22).
- For *practicing physicians*, increasing computerization of practice leaves little time and less opportunity to see their patients in person, resulting in decrease in their confidence in seeing patients. This causes frustration, and has been blamed as one of the causes of *increasing burnout* in physicians in the U.S.
- The main merits of the desktop method are the convenience, the massive data storage and instant analysis of the stored data. But, the students miss the opportunity of learning clinical medicine.
- **e-learning:** In this method, a laptop or an i-pad is uploaded with the information which the students must know and which they can carry about with them, and read and re-read it at their convenience. It is a great thing as a supplement to learning the skills of history taking and physical examination, especially the latter, the hard way, many of which are technique-dependant (see later) and bear repeated viewing. It can supplement bedside teaching but cannot replace it. The modern smart-phone can do the same thing, only better.

History taking, physical examination and thoughtful analysis of the collected data are the three pillars of clinical medicine. Laboratory and imaging data are need-oriented and should be undertaken after a clinical examination, and not instead of them, at least in most instances. However, the laboratorty and imaging data may sometimes be required immediately in seriously ill patients who need prompt treatment.

Symptoms and history taking: What the patient complains of is called **symptoms**. They are the subjective feelings in the patient due to a disease, and which the patient alone can appreciate and narrate its detail to the physician e.g. pain, dyspnoea, nausea, giddiness, thirst, hunger, dizziness, and so on. They have no physical existence and cannot be perceived by the physician or a medical student by using their sense organs viz. touch, vision, hearing and smell. They have to be appreciated by the physician by applying his own mind and experience. They are **physically unverifiable symptoms**. They are like electricity and breeze, which you cannot touch, see or hear; but you can experience their effects such as a lighted electric bulb, a wafted fragrance or rustling of leaves.

Although nobody except the patient can describe exactly the details of his symptoms, sometimes others (family members or friends) may have been told about the details of the symptoms by the patient; or the latter may have observed the consequences of pain such as the patient groaning, crying, turning and twisting in the bed, or the patient may be unconscious. Such a witness can then narrate them to the physician. **Even then, they are called symptoms**. Some of them are **potentially, physically verifiable** (lump, wound, ulcer, bleeding) but have not yet been verified, and are still called symptoms. They are **called physical signs only after they are physically verified by a physician or a medical student. Till then they are symptoms.**

An organized collection of symptoms in a patient constitutes **history**. It may be obtained from the patient, a family member or a friend to whom it has been narrated by the patient, a referral letter from another physician, or past documents if they are available. Pain is a common complaint which brings a patient to the physician, and its analysis serves as the prototype for analysis of many other symptoms.

For the purpose of recording, the history is divided structurally into chief complaint, other symptoms (companion symptoms), history of past illnesses and so on. For details, see chapters on history taking.

Physical signs are the objective evidence of disease **already verified on physical examination** by a physician or by a medical student e.g. fever, a lump, rhonchi, brisk jerks and so on. Some physical signs are easy to verify/elicit/teach e.g. anemia, jaundice, cyanosis (non-technique-dependent signs). Others are technique-dependent, and must be taught formally by a teacher. Examples are examination of the heart, lungs, liver, spleen, central nervous system and so on.

The physical signs, and less often symptoms, are classified as either **hard** or **soft**. These adjectives are used to indicate the **weight** they can add to the interpretation of a physical sign or a symptom obtained during the clinical examination. Most authors reserve these adjectives for physical signs. A few apply them to symptoms as well (Hutchison's Clinical Methods, 23rd edition).

- ***A physical sign is called hard*** if it occurs in a few conditions only, and the clinicians are able to agree upon its presence or absence in a given patient. It adds diagnostic weight to that physical sign in that condition e. g. an extensor plantar reflex.
- ***It is called soft*** if it is known to occur in many different conditions or if the clinicians cannot agree upon its presence or absence in a given patient. It may not add diagnostic weight to that sign in that condition e.g. a soft systolic heart murmur.

- ***A symptom is called hard***, if it is described by many/ most patients in a consistent manner e.g. a rigor (malaria, or a severe, acute infection such as U.T.I.); or tongue biting associated with a seizure (grand mal seizure); and it occurs in a few conditions only.
- ***It is called soft*** if patients describe it variably, especially if asked to repeat the description; or if it is known to occur in many different conditions e.g. dizziness. It has little or no diagnostic weight.

Physical examination is a *ritual* of examination, by a physician or a medical student, of the patient's body for the purpose of eliciting abnormal physical signs as well as confirming what is normal in him. Sometimes, a person with abnormal physical signs may not be aware of them and has no complaints (i.e. symptoms). Such persons are said to be asymptomatic. This happens commonly in conditions such as hypertension.

The physical examination employs several techniques such as Inspection; Palpation; Percussion; Auscultation; Hearing; Smell; Trans-illumination; Succussion splash; Measurement and others. The C.N.S. is examined by using a special protocol of techniques such as testing for muscle strength and tone, sensation, testing for tendon reflexes, and others.

The physical examination is conventionally divided into:

- **General examination**, carried out by the doctor from the moment a patient comes within his view. Its technique is mainly observation. See Chapter 22 for a more detailed explanation.
- **Regional examination**: Thyroid, Breast, a Hernia, Lymph nodes and so on.
- **Examination of organ systems** such as the Respiratory system (R.S.); the Cardiovascular system (C.V.S.); the

Alimentary system (A.S.) and the Central nervous systems (C.N.S.).

Organization and analysis of the collected data is the third pillar of clinical medicine. It is recommended that whereas you should keep your eyes and ears wide open while collecting the data, after it has been collected you should shut your eyes for a while and mull over the data. The data may either fit a clinical picture that you have learnt from a book or shown/taught in the past; this is called pattern recognition. Or, the data may have to be analyzed logically step by step to arrive at a diagnosis, analytic reasoning,

The longer your experience as a practicing clinician, the oftener will the diagnosis fall into the category of pattern recognition. Even so, be wary of spot/instant diagnosis routinely, as it may let you down sometimes. Therefore, even if the diagnosis is obvious, go through the ritual of physical examination from 'head to toe', at least during your trainee years.

Two sides of a coin: Symptoms and abnormal physical signs are the two sides of a coin, an expression of a disturbance in the milieu interior of the body. Symptoms warn the sufferer about a physiological disturbance in the body; and the abnormal physical signs tell the examining doctor about the possible anatomical location of the lesion which caused the symptoms.

Symptoms and physical signs are, therefore, manifestations of two sides of a diseased state in the body. Symptoms and physical signs uncommonly occur singly; they commonly occur in groups of different kinds:

- Asymptomatic e.g. hypertension may be detected by chance during physical examination of a patient.
- Monosymptomatic i.e. a single symptom or sign or a predominant symptom or alone such as in the early

stages of some diseases e.g. static tremor at rest in Parkinson's disease whereas the other physical signs are either minimal or absent.

- A typical combination of symptoms and signs e. g. weight loss in spite of increased appetite, which is highly suggestive of either diabetes mellitus or hyperthyroidism. In most other illnesses, weight loss occurs as a result of decreased appetite due to a the disease.
- Atypical symptom(s) e.g. onset of acute myocardial infarction not with precordial pain but with shortness of breath, or with pain in a less common site such as the lower jaw or interscapular region.
- A characteristic sequence of symptoms and signs as in acute appendicitis: generalized vague abdominal pain, followed by pain and tenderness in the right iliac fossa, and then fever.

Learning history taking and physical examination: There is a major difference between learning the two.

- **Learning history taking**: For this, you need a reasonable command over the language which the patient understands, and over English so that, once you have learnt the basics of history taking, you can advance your knowledge by reading books on your own.
- **Learning physical signs**: There are two types of physical signs, the non-technique-dependent and the technique-dependent. For both, you need a good teacher. He has to **point out** to you the non-technique-dependent signs (such as jaundice, anemia, clubbing and so on), preferably repeatedly on the ward

rounds. He has to demonstrate to you the elicitation of technique-dependent signs (such as those in the R.S., C.V.S., A.S., C.N.S. and many others), and then get you to demonstrate them correctly in his presence. If you have access to an I-pad loaded with video **demonstrations**, you can view them repeatedly at your convenience. No amount of reading a book or hearing a verbal description of the technique will make you good at it. Examples are the ankle jerk and the papillary signs.

Investigations: These should be dictated by the outcome of history and physical examination, at least in most instances. The modern laboratory and imaging tests may help in confirming the clinical diagnosis (e.g. typhoid fever), pinpointing the lesion anatomically (e.g. a pituitary microadenoma); or suggesting an alternative diagnosis. They, either imaging or from the laboratory, have such a high diagnostic accuracy (D.A.) that it is tempting to bypass the history and physical examination and go straight to these tests. That is bad medicine because what a test tells you may be considered often as occurring at a point in time, whereas the evolution of the history and physical examination helps you to build up the natural history of the patient's illness, which is very important.

Chapter 8

Importance of Clinical Medicine

The most important innovation in medicine to come in the next 10 years: the power of the human hand (Abraham Verghese in *A Doctor's Touch*).

Advantages of History Taking and Physical Examination

Harrison's Principles of Internal Medicine, 19th edition, states on page 1, Chapter 1 of the book as follows: "Deductive reasoning and applied technology form the foundation for solution to many clinical problems...yet skill in the most sophisticated applications of laboratory technology and in the use of the latest therapeutic modality alone does not make a good physician" (Quoted verbatim). Braunwald uses similar words in his writings.

Talking to the patient and hearing him out patiently help the physician to establish a rapport with him. The patient feels that the doctor is really interested in him, and he will tell the doctor his problems frankly and without shame or fear. Further, he is more likely to adhere to the doctor's instructions and comply with the prescription.

- He alone can tell you what his most important complaint, chief complaint is, and what has made him come to see you at a particular time.
- The patient can be interviewed and examined on 'as is, where is' basis, and at least a working diagnosis can be reached soon.
- It allows the physician to make an on-the-spot judgment about the patient's credibility by observing not only

what the patient says but how he says it, his demeanor and body language.

- In an acutely or seriously ill patient, the seasoned physician can detect small changes in the patient's condition such as impaired/improved consciousness or cognition during a clinical examination (clinical acumen). This may happen even when the patient's test results are unhelpful.
- In such patients and in children, there is no substitute for the experienced clinician's sixth sense or a 'gut feeling' to judge the seriousness of the illness, beyond what the standard history and physical examination indicate.
- Clinical medicine is learnt primarily by watching and imitating a capable mentor and not from the books and lectures alone. Hence, it is a privilege to be attached to a good teacher during the clinical clerking years.
- The switch over to the electronic, multiple choice system and absence of insistence on the student demonstrating his competence in taking a good history and in carrying out a thorough physical examination, have contributed to the poor ability of the students in developing clinical competence. Unfortunately, a recent paper from the US has stated that the 'in-absence-of-the-patient' method of examining the students is more cost-effective and therefore more acceptable than the old, Oslerian clinical method.
- It may allow on the spot recognition of conditions like Parkinsonism and Down's syndrome, and recognition of dehydration, heart failure, mildly impaired cognition, and a distressed patient.

- A good clinical assessment can limit the number of sophisticated 'tests' to those which are relevant and are likely to provide the maximum diagnostic information in a cost-effective manner.
- There are medical conditions for which there are no established super-test (U.S.G., C.T., M.R.I. and others) criteria; their diagnosis is still by history and physical examination. Some of these conditions are: cellulitis, psoriasis, herpes zoster, amyotrophic lateral sclerosis, Parkinson disease, Bell's palsy, Diabetic retinopathy and others (McGee).
- Therapeutic value of listening to the patient: if you give a patient with a serious, chronic illness, such as an incurable cancer, your time and listen to him, the fact that he is sharing his problems, fears and concerns with you, his doctor, is itself soothing and therapeutic.

Just as the empathetic History Taking can help to create a bond with the patient, so can the thorough physical examination, for an important part of the physical examination is the reassuring and healing touch of the physician's hand (Abraham Verghese and Mosby's book).

Burden of Excessive Dependence on Tests

- Most modern tests are expensive.
- The expenses are not re-imbursed by many insurance companies; and the financial burden of excessive testing is borne by the patient and his family.
- Tests such as repeated C.T. scans can deliver more than permissible amounts of radiation. And, an M.R.I. contrast (gadolinium, now obsolete) can cause a generalized dermopathy in patients with chronic kidney disease.

- Even mildly deviant result of a laboratory or imaging test report may cause avoidable anxiety to the patient and the family.
- Tests may consume time which could be used for initiating therapy, especially in emergencies.
- When you do a lot of tests on a patient, the probability of finding one abnormal result is 1:20 (1 test abnormal out of 20 tests done), purely by chance. Alvan Feinstein has said in his book **Clinical Biostatistics** "In fact, a cynic has said that a normal a person is one who has not had enough tests done on him".

Having said that, it is true that the modern technology is a god-sent boon to us, the human beings. It is also true that the fear of medico-legal problems can lead to defensive practice of medicine and excessive testing by the doctor to save his own back. Therefore, tests should not be shunned but be ordered judiciously and in the best interest of the patient. Before you order a test, especially an expensive or potentially harmful one, you should know why you are asking for the test, and what you will do with its result.

Whatever your specialty, from family practice to cardiac/neuro-surgery, **there is no substitute for an excellent record of detailed history and a thorough physical examination**. Now is the right time for you to learn and start practicing them; for, 'Writing makes an exact man' (Francis Bacon). So, girdle up your waist and start immediately. Remember that the written records of patients treated by Harvey Cushing, a pioneer of neurosurgery over 100 years ago, adorn today the bookshelves of the library of the Peter Bent Brigham Hospital (now, Brigham and Women's Hospital) in Boston, US.

Finally, I urge all of you to read on the internet the following tragic story (The Vanishing Art of Clinical Science-Hyposkillia) by Dr. Anisha Sawkar-Tandon, a radiologist in Bangalore. It will tell you the serious consequences of neglect of history taking and physical examination. It is a must-read story. The path on the internet is: Open Google homepage > Enter the search term 'Vanishing Art of Clinical Science-Hyposkilia by Anisha Sawkar-Tandon' > Click search> Click the website which has the same, complete, above-mentioned search term as the title. The story is displayed.

The following is an exactly opposite story: Ten Minute Miracle by Melissa Zhu Murphy in *Pulse Magazine*, October, 2, 2015. You can read it in the magazine or on the internet. The internet Google path is direct.

Chapter 9

History Taking, Introduction

Let me take the history and I will accept any good intern's word on the physical signs (from the preface to Mcbryde's 'Signs and Symptoms').

We have already seen the difference between symptoms and signs in Chapter 7. Now, we shall learn the method of taking a good history.

We were taught that a good history by itself helped to make a correct diagnosis in 80 per cent of the cases. The veracity of that teaching was always in question.

Quoting the work done in Israel and published by ACP Hospitalists and American College of Physicians in the US in 2014, the latter say that the researchers had found as follows: in internal medicine patients, in whom an emergency and a life threatening disease had been ruled out

(1) History alone helped to make the correct admission diagnosis in 20 per cent of cases. (2) History + physical examination helped in 60 per cent of cases. (3) History + physical examination + the results of routine, simple lab tests +/- E.C.G and +/- X'ray of the of chest helped to make correct diagnosis in 80 per cent - 85 per cent of cases.

History

There are several types of history. They differ from one another mainly in the degree of detail. Each type has its preferred use. The first type, Comprehensive History, is the procedure for taking a detailed history from a patient who has symptoms but not an emergency problem such as severe chest pain or acute abdominal pain. Even in the latter cases, the history of the apparently involved system must be as detailed as the patient and his family can give.

The comprehensive history: This is the mother of all types of history and it records every detail of the patient's current illness, past illnesses, life style, family and socio-economic status and so on. It is primarily for the medical student who must write it in every patient, in order to get used to history taking and recording it. Later on, it may not be necessary in every patient. As your experience grows, you may prune the history taking to suit each patient's requirement. But, certain core items such as the identifying information in detail are a must at all stages of medical practice, as they may have medico-legal implications at any time in future. Comprehensive history is also useful when the patient is being seen for the first time, as it provides the basis for all future assessments. This type of history is possible only in non-emergency (cold), adult cases with internal medicine problems. In pediatric and geriatric patients, in pregnant women, and in patients with emergency or specialty problems, the details of the method have to be modified and trimmed to suit the occasion, although the basic pattern remains the same.

The iterative history: In this type of history, if an experienced and busy physician gets an important clue to the likely diagnosis from what the patient has said thus far, he may ask questions limited and adapted to rule-in or rule-out one possible diagnosis after another until the diagnosis or the most likely diagnosis is reached.

The inventory (multi-session) history: In this type, the history may be taken and recorded in more than one session. In each session, the physician may cover only a part of the patient's story. But, ultimately it emerges as a comprehensive history. This may be necessary when it is expected that the history taking is going to take much longer time than is convenient for either the physician or the patient.

The problem oriented (focussed) history: This type is necessary when the patient's problem appears acute, serious, and possibly life threatening, and needs prompt treatment; examples of such problems are head injury, acute myocardial infarction and acute abdomen.

The interim (i.e. follow up) history: This is history of how the patient has fared since he met you last. This is especially necessary in a patient with a long-standing, chronic disease such as diabetes mellitus or rheumatoid arthritis.

Sources of information: The sources of information are numerous. Information about the patient's illness may obtained from: the Patient himself; Family members; Close friends; patient's chosen **Support person** (Chapter 15) if there is one; even a Passer by in acute episodes; Nurses in the ward; specially Trained social workers; other Physicians and Hospitals that may have treated him in the past; and Past medical records. The contactability of the source of information is precious and should be recorded; and the history should be retrievable quickly. The computerization of medical practice has made that easier.

The history is obtained stepwise. The first item is to verify the identifying information, if it is already entered into the history sheet. After that, spend a few minutes in small talk, getting to know the patient. Thereby, you put him at ease and gain his confidence; he will then be willing to confide his problems to you. Always address the patient by his proper name, even in a busy, public, teaching hospital. Speak to him respectfully. But, insist on as precise information as possible. This requires patience and tact; but it pays in the end.

Read carefully the referral letter if the patient has brought one. Ask him what ails him, what really brings him to meet you, or why he went to his family doctor (if he has one) in the first instance. Do not ask him leading questions which suggest their own answers. Ask open-ended questions. For example, do not ask "Are you getting pain in the stomach". Ask "Do you have any discomfort", which is an open-ended question. That method allows the patient to tell whatever he wishes to tell you, and that too in his own way and in his own words. On his answering "Yes", ask him "What is the nature of the discomfort?" On his answering "Pain" ask him "where?" And, so on. Ask a patient with a chronic illness, why he is seeking your advice at a particular time. Is this the first time he is seeing a doctor for his chronic problem? Is his problem worsening? Has an additional new problem arisen? Is he seeking a second opinion from you? Give him a chance to narrate his problems in his own words.

At this stage, allow the patient to do most of the talking. Avoid interrupting him frequently. Ask him to narrate the story of *his illness* and his concerns (see Chapter 12) about it, in his own words. Although the history is recorded in a standard format, it is neither possible nor advisable to bind the patient to such a rigid format while he is talking. Make brief notes from what he says. They will be useful in getting details from him and when compiling a neat and accurate account in a standard format. But, do not lose eye contact with him by trying to write down everything he says.

If the patient is hard of hearing, confused, stuporous, aphasic, dysarthric, a child, or does not follow the language you speak, there may be genuine difficulty in obtaining the history from him. A similar difficulty may be faced with a patient who is in acute agony. In such cases, the history may have to be obtained from a relative or a friend. In psychiatric patients, a specially trained social worker may have to interview the patient and his relatives for a proper history. On the other hand, in certain circumstances, it may be advisable or even necessary to verify the patient's statements by questioning a relative or a friend. In the case of an epileptic, a description of the seizure will have to be obtained from an eyewitness. If the patient's symptom is brought on by some activity, reproduce that symptom in your presence in your clinic e.g. dizziness brought on by turning the head in a particular direction or pain brought on by walking a certain distance.

The classic example of a disease, where the family members and friends complain that the patient forgets things and events, but the patient is not aware of anything being wrong with him, is Alzheimer's dementia. The patient has no insight into *his illness*. Ascertain whether he really forgets things for good, whether there is only a delay in recall, or perhaps he needs a clue or a hint to jog his memory. Only forgetting for good is consistent with a dementia. Otherwise, it can be simple forgetfulness in the elderly.

The patient may tell you that he has hypertension or a peptic ulcer. Do not accept these diagnostic labels uncritically. Insist gently but firmly on knowing what exactly the patient's complaints are; or else establish and record that he is asymptomatic, but an abnormality has been found by a relative, a friend, by a doctor (e.g. hypertension is found during a routine check up or during examination for an unrelated illness); or he has been detected to have anemia or high blood sugar during laboratory testing. This is important because symptoms may start after the patient comes to know that he has some abnormality. We often see this also in patients with a goiter, who may start worrying after its discovery.

Do not be satisfied with the patient's statement that he feels constipated or dizzy or that he has indigestion. These are layman's terms and are used by different people to mean different things. Try to find out what the patient actually feels e.g. whether he sees a blackout before his eyes (pre-syncope), feels a vague sensation of movement (not amounting to true vertigo); he is unsteady on his feet (dizziness); or he has clear-cut sensation of himself or surroundings spinning (true vertigo).

Different patients may pose different problems during history taking. Some patients are good at giving a coherent account of their illness; others are not. Some are transparent in their answers to your questions; others are evasive because of embarrassment or outright shame at the problem being psychiatric, sex related or financial. Some patients think that a physical illness is respectable, but a psychiatric illness is not. Some patients fear that doctor will diagnose cancer; they are not mentally prepared for it. They may not say anything which, they think, may lead to the diagnosis of cancer. Such patients should be referred to a cancer specialist: e.g. a patient with a supraclavicular lymph node (there is a high chance that it may be metastatic malignancy). Or else, if there is no evidence of cancer, reassure the patient to that effect in clear words. On the other hand, some patients come to you with pages full of written down multiple, somatic complaints in minute detail. Such patients may even come with printouts of information from the internet. There are some patients who would like to please the doctor and they give answers which, they think, he expects. If what the patient says appears inconsistent with the reality, be on the lookout for a psychiatric ailment leading to confabulation, hallucinations or delusions.

Finally, a rare patient may be lying deliberately with an ulterior motive such as financial gain e. g. obtaining false medical bills; or even worse, presenting a false identity or a false alibi. Beware of such patients. Recently, a practicing physician in Mumbai has started photographing every new patient with the web cam and saving the image on the hard disk. This helps the doctor, should the patient present himself or be brought in future with a false identity (changed name) or false alibi.

Chapter 10

Present Illness

A doctor who cannot take a good history and a patient who cannot give one are in danger of giving and receiving bad treatment (Anonymous).

A patient may come with a discrete, single complaint such as a goiter, or bleeding per rectum or breathlessness. Some one else may come with multiple complaints related to one organ system, or to two or more organ systems. In the latter instance, the physician has to help the patient to decide which complaint really made him seek medical advice. Whichever complaint makes the patient seek medical advice is called the **Chief Complaint**. Over and above the chief complaint, he may have ***other (companion) complaints*** too. Do not undervalue the other complaints because one of them may turn out to be more serious than the putative chief complaint. A complaint is a complaint. Pay equal attention to all.

Chief complaint, also called presenting symptom: It is ***the*** reason for the patient's coming to see the doctor. It is narrated by the patient to the doctor in his own words. The patient should be encouraged with such words and phrases as 'would you like to add anything else?' until he says 'No'. Then, record the complaints in a chronological order, meaning the order in which they appeared. The importance of the order of symptoms will be discussed later. If the patient cannot narrate the history in a chronological order, the doctor has to sort it out from the patient's talk and record the complaints as under:

Cough	: 1 month
Fever	: 2 weeks
Blood-stained sputum	: 1 day

Onset, duration and progression: Ask the patient how long he has been unwell (duration of illness). Ask him when the **first symptom** of his present illness started. If there are several complaints, ascertain how long each complaint has existed. Be careful not to accept his first answer to this question without probing further into whether he did or did not have a particular symptom longer than his first answer suggests. *Ask the patient when he was well and in good health last*; and record the answer.

Now, take the complaints one by one and ask the patient to elaborate on the onset and progression of each of them until the present day. After he has finished describing the details of each symptom, ask him further questions to elicit more details, if any. At this stage, too, of eliciting the basic facts, do not ask the patient leading questions.

Ask him whether he noticed his illness himself or it was noticed by someone else and then pointed out to him. Sometimes, the symptoms may start after the patient comes to know that he has an abnormality.

Ask the patient how the illness began **(mode of onset)**. Ask him if he recollects the circumstances in which it began. The best way to judge the onset of an illness is to ask the patient whether he recalls the moment, the hour, the day, the week, the month or even the year when, he thinks, the illness began. The onset may be described as instantaneous, stuttering, sudden or insidious (increasingly longer interval of time from first moment of the illness and of each symptom to its peak intensity). Thus, the rapidity with which the illness progresses from its first moment to its peak can be used to decide the type of its onset.

Onset

Instantaneous (like a bolt from the blue), maximum at the onset of the first symptom.

It occurs

- ***In mechanical defects*** such as a fracture, rupture of muscle fibres, rupture of a sub-pleural bulla to produce pneumothorax and of an intracranial aneurysm to produce sub-arachnoid hemorrhage; and in torsion of a testis;
- ***In arterial or venous embolism***; and
- ***In conditions due to an abnormal electrical discharge*** such as epilepsy, trigeminal neuralgia and paroxysmal tachycardia

Stuttering: It is called stuttering when the illness appears to be gradually and continuously becoming worse; but in fact it is progressing by repetitive additions of worsening as in cerebral thrombotic strokes, or in slow leak from an abdominal organ.

Sudden: Sudden onset occurs quickly, unexpectedly and without warning symptoms, in minute to hours, as in acute infections such as pneumonia.

- ***Sudden onset with a rigor*** occurs in malaria and acute urinary tract infection.

Insidious: The onset is insidious (slow) when from the first moment to the peak of illness takes days to weeks or longer as in chronic infections such as tuberculosis, neurodegenerative, metabolic-endocrine conditions and in neoplastic disorders.

Duration: Try to confirm the duration of the illness and of each symptom.

Progression (time course): The illness may progress in one of the several ways:

- It may progress **rapidly** to its maximum intensity and then may abate to **end in partial or complete**

recovery (as in acute trauma or infection) or end **in death** (myocardial infarction).

- It may progress **gradually but relentlessly** with added episodes of acute illness (chronic bronchitis, degenerative C.N.S. disease).
- It may **worsen** gradually but may show temporary abatements (as in obstructive jaundice due to papillary cholangiocarcinoma i.e. bile duct carcinoma).
- It may be a **lifelong non-progressive state** of mildly substandard health (thalassemia trait).
- It may consist of **repetitions of transient events** (epilepsy, migraine, vertigo, colic or syncope) or **not-so-transient events** (disseminated sclerosis) with complete or almost complete remission between the episodes.
- It may show classic **periodicity** as in peptic ulcer i.e. there may be symptomatic periods of weeks, separated by symptom-free intervals of months.

The onset, duration and mode of progression of an illness, constitute its '**natural history**'. Delineation of the natural history of an illness helps in making a diagnosis. An organ or an organ system may be capable of responding to an offending agent in a limited number of ways. Hence, the symptoms arising from an organ or an organ-system may be relatively few, and are likely to be common to most diseases involving that organ or organ-system. Moreover, some symptoms (e.g. dyspnoea) occur in more than one body-system; and, the disease may be in any of two or more systems such as lungs and heart. Therefore, it is the **combination** of symptoms, their order of appearance, and the **natural history** of the illness that help to make clinical diagnosis.

With febrile illnesses, a lot of importance used to be attached to the **shape of the graph of the fever** e.g. continuous, intermittent, remittent, relapsing and so on. In more recent times, these attributes of fever have ceased to be useful in making a diagnosis with confidence. This is partly because of the practice of starting an antimalarial drug or an antibiotic expectantly before the cause of fever is ascertained. **Exceptions** to these statements are: (a) in tropical countries, the presence of a 'stepladder', remittent fever is highly specific for typhoid fever; and (b) relative bradycardia is still thought to be consistent with the diagnosis of typhoid fever, dengue fever and other viral infections (McGee).

Sensitive issues: Patients may be embarrassed to discuss with the physician certain issues. They can be called *sensitive issues.* Examples are numerous: Putative Psychiatric illness; Financial concerns; Physical deformities; Alcohol consumption; Drug abuse; certain sexual practices; Dying or death of a loved one; Unpleasant family interactions such as spouses not getting on with each other; Parents not getting on with their grown up and earning children; Domestic violence; Bowel or urinary incontinence; H.I.V.; and more. The physician should broach these topics only after establishing a rapport with the patient, perhaps after the physical examination; and that too after gently explaining to him the need for such discussion on one or more of these problems. Be non-judgmental during the discussion and assure the patient of the confidentiality of the information revealed by him.

Currently used drugs: The patient should be asked whether he is currently taking any drugs (modern medicine drugs, complementary drug therapy or alternative drug therapy); are they physician-prescribed or self-prescribed? An over-the-counter (O T C) drug for any ailment? What is patient's response to it? Has the initial, beneficial response continued, diminished or ceased (*Drug failure*)?

He should also be asked about habitual consumption of strong coffee, tobacco in any form, alcohol and recreational drugs, either *therapeutic* (legal) drugs such as psychotropic drugs; or street (illegal) drugs i.e. drugs of abuse such as opium, cannabis, ketamine and so on and so forth.

Ask him whether he was on any drug(s) shortly before the present illness started (*Drug intolerance or drug allergy*). Is he being treated with multiple drugs (*polypharmacy*) and may be suffering from drug-drug interaction? The last query is important especially in the elderly because polypharmacy is frequent in them.

Ask the patient to bring all drugs he is taking for you to see.

Chapter 11

Diet and Physiological Functions

To read without reflecting is like eating without digesting (Edmund Burke).

Dietary history: The students should try to learn from the institution's dietician how to obtain a patient's dietary history, and then make an attempt to obtain one, although they may have to refer the patient to the dietician for a detailed diet history.

Measure the patient's height and weight and calculate his B.M.I. (see Chapter 23).

(1) Ask the patient how many meals he eats per day. Are his meal times constant? How often does he eat out? Obtain from the patient the approximate daily quantities of different food items, (rice, rotis, dal, raw salads, leafy and tuberous vegetables, fruits, milk, eggs and meat) he consumes daily in terms of numbers (fruits and eggs) and approximate number of cups of cooked foods. Enquire about: (a) *Salt and sugar* consumption (low, moderate or high), (b) About consumption of sweets (fat and sugar), (c) *Aerated sweet drinks* (sugar), (d) *Nuts*, and (e) *Commercially available fried snacks* (trance fatty acids—T.F.A in this case). Enquire about family members and the amounts of oil, *ghee and butter* consumed by the family per month. (e) Enquire about alcohol consumption: type, quantity, frequency and how long he has been consuming it.

(b) Enquire about the intake of water, especially in the elderly; they may not be drinking enough water, and are prone to develop dehydration.

(c) If the patient on a multivitamin pill, check the composition of the pill. Always keep in mind Vitamin D deficiency especially in the elderly, and Iron deficiency in women of the reproductive age.

(d) Enquire also about the patient's lifestyle and physical activity e.g. Walking, Gyming, Swimming, etc, or whether he has a sedentary lifestyle. How long per day does he sit at his office table and his home working table?

Remember that obesity is as much malnutrition as under-nourishment with weight loss and vitamin deficiencies is.

Physiological functions: The following physiological functions should be enquired into. Special attention should be paid to a recent change in any of them.

In Males and Females

(1) Sleep: Is it adequate (requirement is variable; the optimum is 6-8 hours nightly in adults;), and refreshing? Is it disturbed? If so, the reason (pain, discomfort, dyspnoea, polyuria, anxiety, sleep apnoea, working late into night (Don't; **Goodnight. Sleep Clean**),** or no apparent reason. Insomnia is difficulty in falling asleep; or awakening very early or frequently. Is there reversal of sleep rhythm with drowsiness or compulsive sleep during daytime along with insomnia at night? Is any hypnotic drug being taken currently?

This has reference to an article which stresses the importance of **adequate, sound sleep (6 hours, at a minimum) every night in adults. The title is "Further Reading in Glymphatic System" by Wikipedia. It is on the internet. One line summary is 'The tired, daytime-awake brain cleanses itself of the harmful, accumulated, metabolic waste only during sound sleep at night'.

Follow this practice if you want your health and mental faculties to remain in good condition.

(2) Appetite: Good; excessive; poor—for all foods or certain foods only? Does the patient know the reason? Has he always been a small/hefty eater? Does he enjoy the meals and is looking forward to them? Or does he eat because it is mealtime? Does he miss a meal because of the abdominal discomfort/pain after eating? Alternatively, has the appetite increased (diabetes mellitus and thyrotoxicosis)?

(3) Thirst: Decreased (especially in the elderly); Increased (in summer and in dehydration); for Chilled water (diabetes insipidus).

(4) Micturition (urination): Frequency D/N, increased more than once at night (nocturia); Volume (normal volume depends on the fluid intake); Scanty (oliguria—less than 25 ml/hour for four hours, or less than 500 ml/24 hours; it commonly occurs because of drinking insufficient water. So, ask him how many glasses of water he generally drinks per day). Oliguria is also a symptom diminished extracellular fluid volume. Copious (polyuria); Increased frequency without polyuria (UTI). Blood in urine. Pain supra-pubic or in the loin. Burning during urination; Has to Strain; is there Urgency; Precipitancy; Incontinence; Hesitancy? Size of urinary Stream? History of passing urinary Stone(s).

(5) Bowels: Frequency (maximum three times a day to at least once in three days minimum is considered as normal); Consistency (well formed, unformed, watery, hard); Constipation (infrequent or hard-to-pass stools); Diarrhoea (frequent, unformed or watery stools). Colour (normal, dark, pale); Blood (digested or frank blood); Melena (black tarry stools associated with gastro-intestinal bleeding); Mucus; Pus; Associated Pain (before, during or after defecation); Flatulence; Is the Pain relieved by defecation? Borborygm; Habitual use of laxatives or enemas?

(6) Sweating: Is it at the level customary with the patient? Increased? Decreased? Ask about Heat tolerance, Cold tolerance. Feels Feverish?

In Females

(7) Menstrual history: (a) Age at *Menarche* (first menstrual period)? (b) Age at *Menopause* define as absence of menstrual period for 12 months since the last one? (c) Periods regular? 5/30 indicates bleeding for 5 days and cycle of 30 days (from first day of one period to the fist day of the next period). Normal cycle is 24-35 days. (d) *Periods* moderate, excessive, scanty by subjective assessment; (e) *Amenorrhoea* is missing three successive periods in the absence of pregnancy. (f) Past menstrual history? (g) *Last menstrual* period (L.M.P.)? (h) *Contraception* practiced? What method?

(8) Obstetric history: (a) Total number of pregnancies (*Gravidity* = *G*)? (b) Number of deliveries viz. live births and stillbirths, at twenty weeks or longer duration; (Parity=P)? For example G4/P3; (c) Miscarriges: Spontaneous expulsion of the fetus before it becomes viable by 20 weeks? Most miscarriages occur by 14 weeks (d) Antepartum hemorrhage (A.P.H.)? (e) Postpartum hemorrhage (P.P.H.). (f) State of health during pregnancies? Any drug treatment during pregnancies? Details of drug therapy? (g) Was Lactation established even for a short time? Did it never occur? or was it suppressed with drugs? (h) Breast feeding and its duration after each live birth?

Chapter 12

Specific Interrogation, Empathy, Associated Symptoms and Symptom Analysis

Empathy is about standing in someone else's shoes, feeling with his or her heart, seeing with his eyes (Daniel Pink).

Specific Interrogation

Now is the time to ask the patient a number of direct (closed ended, even yes-no) questions to elicit points in the history which he may have forgotten to mention or never even thought of. In certain cases, it may be necessary to ask the patient to observe his own symptoms in a particular way and then come back.

Experienced physicians may decide which part of the history should be pursued further in detail and what part may be left out. But, the beginner must be systematic and thorough, and must not omit any part of history taking.

One further advantage of thorough interrogation is that it establishes a good rapport and permits the physician to know the patient as a human being and not as a case of peptic ulcer. For, it has been said that "There are no diseases; there are only sick people" (Trousseau). And, we should be treating sick people, not diseases.

Empathy: The physician is interested in making a diagnosis in a patient. On the other hand, the patient has concerns about the effects of the illness on his lifestyle e. g. Working capacity, sleep, sexual functioning, the possibility of loss of job and more. The treating physician must understand the patient's concerns as if they were his own. Such understanding by the doctor is possible if he has ever experienced the patient's problems himself, or he can put himself in the patient's shoes and experience mentally the patient's problems; it is called empathy, and it has therapeutic value.

Associated symptoms are those which accompany the chief complaint. Both may arise in the same organ system, and may be causally related. They are helpful as they suggest the possible cause of the chief complaint. For example, nausea and visual flashes are typically associated with classical migraine. A convulsive seizure along with tongue biting suggests the diagnosis of grand mal epilepsy. Rigors along with fever suggest malaria or urinary tract infection. Acne, temporal recession of hair, hisutism and acanthosis nigricans associated with irregular periods suggest the diagnosis of polycystic ovarian syndrome.

Symptom Analysis

Every symptom, whether expressed by the patient on his own (chief complaints and other complaints, Chapter 9) or found during a system symptom review (Chapter 13) should be analyzed thoroughly. This is description of the complaint by the patient in his own words. The same words (dizziness, numbness, blurred vision) may mean different things to different patients. Each physician has a slightly different plan e. g. the order in which the questions are asked. One such plan of symptom analysis follows.

Questionnaire for symptom analysis: Pain being one of the commonest symptoms in clinical practice, the questionnaire below is based on analysis of pain. It acts as a prototype for analysis of most other symptoms, with possibly some modifications. Some authors call such analysis '*The seven attributes of a symptom*'.

- What is troubling you? Please tell me in your own words.

- If it is pain, where is it? At which sites in the body? Where is it maximum? Please point out the site of maximum pain with a finger.
- What type of pain is it? Dull aching, burning, colicky, shooting, stabbing, squeezing, splitting, cramping, nauseating, sickening? Is it exhausting? If the patient cannot respond with one of these adjectives to describe his pain, you may offer him some of these words and ask him to match them with his pain. Even this may be difficult for a non-English-speaking patient.
- Onset, duration and progression: O.D.P. (Chapter 10)? Content or quantity e. g. vomitus, expectoration, blood loss, stool?
- Radiation or movement from one site to another; mostly applies to pain; please indicate with a finger the path of movement.
- Is it continuous or intermittent? If the latter, duration of each episode and the duration of symptom-free intervals? Is it paroxsysmal (abrupt in onset and abrupt in cessation)? What is the frequency of the episodes?
- Intensity and severity: does it interfere with any aspect of lifestyle e.g, appetite, sleep, ability to walk or climb a staircase, office work, playing with children, taking the wife out, sexual activity?
- Precipitating, aggravating and relieving factors? Relation to time of the day and to one or more of the numerous factors, appropriate for the symptom. Some of them are: posture; stance; movement; lying down; activity such as sitting, walking, running, exercise, eating, starving, swallowing, vomiting,

urination, bowel movement, breathing, coughing, season of the year, ambient temperature, straining, manual pressure, menstrual period; exposure to hot sun; drugs; and more?

- Any associated symptoms (see above)?
- Medication and response to it? In some instances the relieving effect of a drug is diagnostic; examples are colchicine in an attack of acute gouty arthritis; quinine in malaria; organic nitrates in angina, and so on? This may be a sort of 'therapeutic trial'.
- Effect of drugs known to be generally effective?
- Any change in the type or severity of a symptom e.g. getting worse, not responding to a drug which was effective to begin with?
- Any new symptom?

Chapter 13

System Symptom Review (S.S.R.)

System Symptom Review (S.S.R.) is *questioning the patient systematically* for possible symptoms from all body systems to detect any problem which may possibly co-exist in a system but is undetected. It is a list of direct, often yes-no (*opposite of indirect and open-ended*) questions, arranged by organ and organ system, designed to uncover any hidden dysfunction or disease. If such direct questions are not asked, some disease condition may be missed. A problem so detected *may sometimes be more serious than the chief complaint and other symptoms* (Chapter 10); and it should be subjected to the same close scrutiny as the chief complaint. Such direct or yes-no questions are *also useful in eliciting past history, family history and personal-social history.*

The questions to be asked under the S.S.R. are listed below organ/system-wise. *The patient's answers are analyzed according to the plan of 'Symptom Analysis'* (Chapter 12). The analysis of all symptoms detected is likely to reveal all the patient's feelings and concerns about his illness. It is always good to ask the patient whether he would like to add anything to whatever he has already told you. This is your opportunity to practise what you learned in Chapter 12. Finally, ask the patient "Do you have any idea about the possible cause of your illness"? He might give you a surprise.

General Health: How are you feeling today? What is the problem? Pain? Fever? Chills? Night sweats? Fatigue (tiredness or weariness, in need of rest or sleep which relieves it)? Fatigability (extreme or prolonged tiredness and decreased capacity for work because of an illness or prolonged overwork)? Usual weight, Involuntary weight change? Weight loss of 5 per cent or more in 6 months should be investigated. Able to cope with life and all the work that is expected of you? Clothes fitting more loosely or more tightly than before? Bleeding—if yes at one site, then bleeding at any other site? Past history of bleeding after minor trauma? Family history of bleeding disorder? Swelling? Lump anywhere? Increase in size of hands and feet (acromegaly)? Wasting (shrinking) anywhere in the body)? History of blood transfusion (possible exposure to infections especially hepatitis B and H.I.V.)?

Skin and its Appendages

Skin: Any skin problem? Dryness; Itching; Rashes; Soreness; Lump; Change in colour (pallor or darkening; yellow palms)? Circumscribed white patches (vitiligo); Generalized absence of skin pigmentation, plus the colourless iris (albinism)? Ask about: Sweating; Acne; Moles; Skin lines (striae).

Hair: Change in quantity and distribution (scalp, eyelashes, eyebrows, beard, armpits, trunk; limbs)? Change in texture (soft/rough/oily)? Patches of complete loss of hair (alopecia areata)? Selective loss of hair (loss of outer ⅓rd of eyebrows in hypothyroidism)? Temporal recession of hair in women? Hirsutism (male type of hair growing in women)? Hypertrichosis (growth of hair in areas excluding those which are androgen dependent in both men and women? Common causes are drugs-phenytoin, minoxidil and acetazolamide).

Nails: Colour: healthy pink; or pale; blue; yellow? Brittle? Change in shape Koilonychia; Platonychia; Clubbing? Diminution in rate of growth (normal 0.1mm/day in finger nails; less in toe nails)?

Head and Associated Organs

Head: Headache? Dizziness (lightheadedness)? Vertigo? Diminished vision? Double vision (diplopia)? Convulsions? Repeated loss of consciousness (epilepsy)? Impairment or loss of vision in entire or partial field of vision (blindness)? Head injury?

Eyes: Colour: Pale (anemia),Yellow (jaundice), Blue (cyanosis); Diminished vision? Long-sighted or short-sighted? Wear glasses (including contact lenses) for reading/distant objects? Pain? Watering? Last eye examination? Need extra light for reading (with advancing age)? Angry redness? Soreness? Itching? Discharge? Dryness (xerophthalmia)? Vision poor in dim light or darkness (night blindness or nyctalopia)? Bitot's spots (both due to Vitamin A deficiency)? Flashes of light? Floaters?

Ear, nose and throat: With a complaint in any one of the three, ask questions about all three.

Ears: Ear ache? Discharge? Fever? Diminished hearing? Vertigo? Tinnitus (hearing a sound without an external stimulus)? Use a hearing aid?

Nose and paranasal sinuses: Cough? Running nose? Blocked nose? Dry nose? Nasal itching? Repeated sneezing? Diminished sense of smell? Epistaxis (nosebleed)? Frequent colds? Are symptoms seasonal or all year round? How long do symptoms last? Foul smell from the nose with loss of ability to smell (atrophic rhinitis)? Pain over sinuses? Frontal headache? Dizziness? Vertigo?

Throat: Sore throat? Pain in the throat? Difficulty in swallowing? Hoarse voice? Blood stained saliva?

Mouth and Related Parts

Lips: Itching? Dryness? Soreness? Swelling?

Mouth: Dry (drinks enough water?) Soreness? Pain? Diminished sense of taste? Food tastes pungent? Chewing tobacco? Smoking?

Tongue: Poor sense of taste? Soreness? Pain? Tongue biting? Movement impaired?

Teeth: All teeth intact/any missing/broken/cavities? Denture? Difficulty in chewing food? Care of teeth (brushing teeth and rinsing mouth)? Holes in the teeth (caries)? Smoking? Chewing tobacco?

Gums: Pain? Bleeding? Pyorrhea? Recession and atrophy? Hypertrophy (phenytoin)?

Throat: See above

Esophagus: Difficulty (dysphagia) or pain (odynophagia) during swallowing? Is the difficulty more for solids or liquid? Point out with a finger where the food sticks.

Neck, Breasts and Axillae

Neck: Pain? Stiffness? Any Lump (goiter, lymph nodes)?

Breasts: Discomfort? Pain? Nipple discharge: serous, milky, blood tinged? Spontaneous or after compression of the nipples? Feel a lump in your breast? Galactorrhoea i. e. inappropriate milk secretion (consumption of certain drugs hypothyroidism, pituitary tumors, fondling of the breasts)? Also see Chapter 4.

Axillae: Odour? Lump? Reduction in or loss of hair? Itching? Boils? Rash? Darkening (deodorants, pregnancy, over-enthusiastic and frequent depilation, Addison's disease)? Hyperpigmentation with coarseness (acanthosis nigricans). Method of hair removal? Deodorant use?

Respiratory System (R.S.): Cough (duration, dry or productive; seasonal or perennial? Precipitating/relieving factors)? Expectoration (sputum: colour, consistency, serous, mucoid, pus, odour; estimated quantity in 24 hours)? Dry cough and moist cough sound different. Smoking (self or anybody at home or workplace)? Environmental dust exposure? Hemoptysis (coughing out blood-tinged, rusty brown sputum or frank red blood? How much)? Dyspnoea (shortness of breath = painless but uncomfortable awareness of breathing, disproportionate to the level of exertion)? Severity—how much exertion brings it on? Does it interfere with lying down on the bed, not necessarily relieved on sitting up; contrast this with orthopnoea of L.V.F. which is relieved by sitting up. Wheezing (whistling sound mostly during expiration; relieved by bronchodilators; may be heard at a short distance from the patient)? Severe difficulty in breathing (due to obstruction in larynx, trachea or bronchi)? Chest pain (pleural; contrast with anginal pain and pain of rib fracture)? History of chest infection (viral, chronic bronchitis, pneumonia)? Has there ever been any allergy anywhere in the body? Travelled recently?)? Exposure to tuberculosis? Last X'ray chest and its report?

Cardiovascular System (C.V.S.): Fatigability (see above)? Known history of rheumatic fever, heart murmur, hypertension? Daily physical activity? Chest pain (angina pectoris i.e. pain in the precordium during exertion)? Palpitation (awareness of the beating of the heart, most often non-cardiac except in cardiac arrhythmias)? Cough (sometimes a symptom of left ventricular failure, L.V.F.)? Dyspnoea? Orthopnoea (dyspnoea on lying down)? Paroxysmal nocturnal dyspnoea (waking up from sleep at night due to dyspnoea; P.N.D.)? Edema (swelling due to accumulation of water) in dependent parts (legs and sacral region); rarely face; uni-or bilateral? Pitting or non-pitting? Hemoptysis? Feeling faint = blacking out (presyncope)? If followed by transient loss of consciousness (syncope)? Oliguria (scanty urine)? Nocturia (increased frequency of urination at night; normal = none or once at night)? How much physical exercise do you take and how long do you sit at your work table daily? Sitting for long hours daily without a break is an independent risk factor for obesity and metabolic syndrome. The risk cannot be countered by exercising during other hours of the day; but it can be countered by NEAT while sitting for long hours (See Chapter 15). Last E.C.G. and its report?

Peripheral vascular system: Hypertension? Intermittent vasculogenic claudication (limping due to pain in the calf muscles on walking, relieved by resting and by standing; differentiate it from neurogenic claudication in which lower limb pain occurs in legs along with pain in back, buttocks and thighs on standing and walking, and is not relieved by standing but is relieved by sitting)? Leg cramps? Pain in the feet and legs (any time; during sleep)? Blackening of toes? Swelling with or without tenderness in the toes? Pain in the calf at rest? Peripheral cyanosis +/- pain in the cyanosed parts? Varicose veins? Thrombophlebitis? Gangrene?

Gastrointestinal System (G.I.S.): Dysphagia? Pain in abdomen—acute or chronic? Appetite? (looking forward to a meal and enjoying it; contrast with hunger – a feeling of discomfort or weakness caused by lack of food, coupled with desire to eat, and relieved by eating). Is it distaste for food or fear of pain in abdomen after eating? Early satiety while eating a meal? Excessive salivation? Indigestion = discomfort on eating? Food intolerance? Heartburn (a burning sensation in the chest caused by regurgitation of gastric contents, either acid or bile, into the esophagus)? Waterbrash = regurgitation of excess accumulated saliva from the lower part of the esophagus. Nausea (the state which precedes vomiting; feeling 'sick')? Vomiting (throwing out forcefully stomach contents involuntarily through mouth and nose)? Hematemesis (vomiting of blood)? Melena (black, "tarry" stools that are associated with gastrointestinal bleeding)? Passing red blood per rectum? Hemorrhoids? Flatulence (flatus expelled through the mouth or anus)? Constipation? Diarrhoea? Yellow eyes? (jaundice); Food habits? what you eat; eat meals at regulars hours?); Eating habit? how you eat, leisurely or hurriedly; gulp food? Feel a lump in the abdomen?

Kidneys and urinary tract: Pain in the loin +/- radiating to groin? Suprapubic pain? Urinary frequency, Urgency, Dysuria? Strangury? Nocturia? Urinary flow abnormality? Polyuria, oliguria, anuria? Fever with rigor? Hematuria? Foul smelling urine? Edema? Nausea-vomiting? Projectile vomiting = forceful vomitting, not preceded the customary nausea? History of passing stone(s)? Family history of passing stones? Known high blood pressure? Lump?

Groins: Mass (lymph nodes); or Hernia (lump on coughing or straining)?

Genitals (female): External genital or pelvic pain? Menstrual and obstetric history (Chapter 11); Amenorrhoea, primay (not having the first period by fourteenth birthday and no beginning of secondary sex characters starting to appear)? Or a sexually mature woman missing three consecutive periods in the absence of pregnancy (secondary)? Vaginal discharge (with or without itching, pain, foul smell)? Intermenstrual or postmenopausal vaginal bleeding? Pain during sexual intercourse (dyspareunia)? Sexual satisfaction? Low or absent sexual libido (libido = sexual desire)? Contraception? Method of contraception?

Genitals (male): Pain in the penis, perineum or scrotum? Irritation and inflammation of the space between glans penis and foreskin (balanitis in uncontrolled diabetes)? Small or diminished size of testes? Urethral discharge? Lump in the scrotum hydrocele? History of a sexually transmitted disease? (sensitive topic, be cautious); Sexual function: sexual desire (libido), frequency of sex, performance (adequate penile erection for vaginal penetration)? Ejaculation and time to it from penile insertion? Sexual satisfaction? Use of condom? Persistent painful erection of penis (priapism).

Musculoskeletal system: Pain +/- tenderness or lump in muscles, joints, bones? Stiffness/swelling of joints? Painful movements and deformity at joints? Backache cervical, dorsal, lumbar)? Fever? Chills? Loss of appetite? Weight loss? Weakness and wasting of muscles? Bone pains? History of fracture especially on minimum trauma?

Endocrine-metabolic system: Known diabetes or its risk factors? Hyperlipidemia? Thyroid disorder (commonly a swelling in the neck, goitre)? Fatigability? Recent weight gain or loss? Cold or heat intolerance? Excessive or diminished sweating-hunger-thirst? Weight loss in spite of increased appetite (diabetes mellitus, thyrotoxicosis)? Neck surgery/radiation? Very severe polyuria and/or craving for chilled water (diabetes insipidus)? Increase in shoe or glove size (acromegaly)? Bone pains? Protruding eyes; Rounding of face? Repeated fractures, especially non-traumatic?

Hematologic system: Pallor (anemia); Fatiguability? Prolonged unexplained fever? Easy bruising? Bleeding? History of transfusion +/- transfusion reaction? Family history of similar illness?

Allergy: See Chapter 17.

Neurologic System (C.N.S.): Headache? Dizziness? Vertigo (a clear-cut description of spinning feeling)? Blackouts? Fainting (passing out)? Diminished muscle strength (paresis)? Complete loss of muscle strength (paralysis)? Muscle cramps? Numbness (diminished ability to feel the sensation)? Tingling? Tremors? Other involuntary movements? Seizures? Difficulty in articulation of speech (dysarthria)? Inability to form speech (aphasia)? Head injury? History of boxing? Stroke? Transient ischemic attacks (T.I.As.)?

Psychiatric: Nervousness? Feeling depressed? Maniacal? Suicidal thoughts? Anxiety? Impaired concentration? Forgetfulness? Impaired cognition (inability to learn) see Chapter 31 for definition? Whether patient complains of forgetfulness, or relatives complain of it whereas patient is unaware of it?

Criticism: There is some criticism of routine, non-selective System Symptom Review (S.S.R.) in every patient: "It is not productive except when done selectively". But, this privilege does apply to students under training. They must do the history completely in every patient in order to learn how to do it properly.

Chapter 14

Past History

The past history is the baseline for assessing the presenting complaints (Mosby).

In this chapter, we enquire about health and illnesses from birth to the present day.

- Birth weight, if known? Low birth weight (less than 2500 g) with catch-up growth is a predictor of metabolic syndrome in later life (Barker).
- Immunizations in childhood, as recommended? Do you have a record of them?
- What was your lifestyle in childhood and adolescence-was it one of plenty or of wants? Was there enough to eat, enough clothing, enough sleep, and adequate medical attention?
- Were you brought up in an atmosphere of love, peace, kindness and friendliness (Tender Loving Care, T.L.C.) or in one of harshness, if not battering?
- Do you remember any one saying that you were growing too slowly at any time?
- What was your school and college performance like? Did you participate in outdoor activities? Did you have friends?
- Were you content with life then?
- Were you brimming with good health? Or, were you falling ill repeatedly? Did you have measles, chicken pox, diphtheria, repeated sore throat,

repeated or prolonged diarrhoea, worms, allergy, injury or accident resulting in disability; a kidney problem? Surgery? Tuberculosis? Rheumatic fever? Any other diagnosed infection? Asthma? Bleeding? Jaundice? Fits? Any illness requiring investigations and/ or prolonged absence from school or college? Prolonged drug treatment? Hospitalization? Transfusion? Vision and Hearing normal or defective? Treatment for the same?

- Did you smoke or consume tobacco in any form? How much and how long? Alcohol? Taken street drugs? At what age did you start it and when did you give it up?
- When did you achieve puberty?
- Did have you any adult illness: Tuberculosis, Hepatitis, Diabetes, Hypertension, Heart disease? Serious infection? Accident? Injury? Worms? Surgery? Hospitalization?
- Did you ever have an illness similar to the present one, in the past?

Some of the above questions must always be asked. For other questions, use your discretion. Nobody can ask all the questions to all patients even if it is supposed to be a comprehensive history. If the answer to any of the above questions is positive, try to go into as much detail as possible, including past records, if available. **Be careful about sensitive issues** while choosing the questions and their wording—say, those about recreational street drugs, or treatment for a sexually transmitted disease such as H.I.V.. Otherwise, you might be accused of impropriety.

Chapter 15

Personal and Social History

The contents of someone's bookcase are part of his history (Anatole Broyard).

- Socio-economic class: Working class (blue collar); middle class (white collar); and affluent class, as judged by job designation, income, residential address, life-style, having one or more car(s).
- Birth; childhood lifestyle; treatment received from parents (loving, friendly, aggressive, dominating)? Education and school-college performance; ability to make friends?
- Do you think you are healthy, happy and feel well? How are appetite, bowels, urination, sleep, job satisfaction, hobbies, reading habit, friends? See WHO definition of 'health' in Chapter 5.
- Have you any long-standing medical illness?
- Dietary pattern and its adequacy; sedentary or physically active?
- Occupation, work place, job designation and description of work (do not accept "I go to office"), work satisfaction and economic satisfaction; exposure to any hazardous substance; transportation to and from work place; habits and leisure time–How do you spend it-with family, friends, reading, hobbies, playing with children, taking wife out, playing or watching games? What are your sources of entertainment and enjoyment?

- Consumption of strong coffee, alcohol, tobacco in any form, street drugs? Go into details (type, quantity, frequency, duration).
- Home conditions, marital status and sexual satisfaction? Children-how are they doing at school?
- Are you the sole earner? Employed or unemployed? What is your income, if you do not mind, please? Access to medical care, its type and affordability; support group (relatives, friends, state, charity)?
- Have to support anybody financially, e.g. parents, chronically ill or disabled family member?
- Any non-medical problem bothering you?
- What precautionary measures do you follow to avoid illness?

Do You

(1) Eat sensibly? Maintain normal body weight i.e. B.M.I. between 18.5 and 24.9?

(2) Indulge in structured physical activity, either

(a) Regular exercise = physical activity such as walking briskly, so that you sweat, for 30 minutes, at least 5 times a week? If you do not sweat you are walking too slowly to get the full benefit; if you feel exhausted at the end of the walk it is too fast. This is applicable to adults aged 18-65 years. (Medscape); or

(b) Non-Exercise-Activity-Thermogenesis (NEAT): "Wiggle your body, stand, walk back and forth while waiting for something or someone, avoid using the elevator, get up and walk for a few minutes in the middle of your work, tap your toes, shop, dance, wet-mop the floor in your house, walk to and back from your workplace" (Mayo Clinic).

A sound advice is that throughout the waking hours of day (1) If you can walk, don't stand, walk; (2) If you can stand, don't sit, stand; (3) If you can sit, don't lie down, sit.

These activities boost your NEAT. Some of these activities are simply fidgeting in common language. They can burn as many as 100 to 800 calories per day. It can be a significant factor in stabilizing weight despite variations in food intake, and they can be modulated consciously. NEAT can counter the risk posed by prolonged sitting for many hours, daily, at the work table (See C.V.S. Chapter 12).

(3) Control diagnosed diseases with lifestyle changes and/or drugs e.g. diabetes mellitus, hypertension, coronary heart disease, vitamin D deficiency?

(4) Have you been immunized as recommended for the elderly (65 years or more): influenza vaccine, pneumococcal vaccine, tetanus vaccine and herpes zoster vaccine, in the US?

(5) Get an annual medical check up (physical examination, fasting blood sugar, LDL cholesterol, colonoscopy, mammography, pelvic examination. The benefit of some of these tests has not yet been documented. There is a lot of debate about the annual medial check up, especially its financial aspects See NEJM 15-10-2015 for pro and cons.

Activities of Daily Living (ADLs) need to be assessed in the elderly (age 65 years and more) and in disabled persons of any age. It tells you how well the patient can look after himself at home, with and without help of others and/or gadgets (functional status). Do you need a support person (an individual hired or chosen to accompany you or a person with a disability to provide services or assistance with communication, mobility, personal care, medical needs or access to goods or services).

The activities commonly assessed are:

Physical activities: Personal hygiene (practices associated with the preservation of health and healthy living); Grooming (the art of cleaning, and maintaining parts of the body and clothing, viz care of hair, teeth, nails, clothes, socks, shoes); Bathing; Dressing and undressing; Self feeding; Getting into and out of bed and wheel chair); Getting on to and off the toilet; Bowel and bladder management (continence); Walking at home with or without a cane, a walker or crutches.

Instrumental activities: Doing housework; Preparing a simple meal; Taking medications as prescribed; Managing money; Shopping for small things; Answering phone; Walking to nearby places.

Chapter 16

Family History

There are only two lasting bequests we can give our children: one is roots, and the other, wings (Hodding S. Carter).

Knowledge of the family history helps to identify a predisposition to develop certain illnesses, and enables you to avoid triggers in the environment.

- Has a relative an illness with features similar to those of your current illness?
- If the disease runs in the family, ask about every one from grandparents to cousins.
- Enquire about the health, known disease, death, age at death and cause of death, if relevant.
- **In first degree relatives,** i. e. parents, children and siblings.
- **In second degree relatives,** i.e. grandparents, grandchildren, aunts, nieces, uncles and nephews; and
- **In third degree relatives:** first cousins.

The list of disease conditions is long, but enquire at least about heart disease, high blood pressure, diabetes, stroke, asthma, and cancer.

P.S.: A massive controlled study (retrospective analysis of records of past 40 years from Scandinavian registries) suggests that if a person's one parent dies before the person's age of 18 years, there is increased (twice) risk of suicide later in life in the bereaved person than in controls, although the actual incidence of suicide is low in both groups. The risk continues for 25 years after the event. Therefore, *enquire in detail about the well being of every patient's parents routinely*. The highly distressed bereaved child, if detected at the time of the event, needs help to cope with the bereavement (Abstract in Physician's First Watch (NEJM) dated 12-11-2015; original article in Online JAMA Psychiatry dated 11-11-2015).

Chapter 17

Allergy and Travel History

Did God who gave us flowers and trees, also provided the allergies? (Yip Harburg).

History of Allergy

- **Allergic symptoms:** The common allergic reactions are: skin rashes, conjunctivitis, rhinitis, bronchospasm, stomach ache, diarrhoea, etc. The most severe reaction is anaphylaxis after injection of penicillin or anti-tetanus horse serum, which can be lethal, unless treated immediately. It is best prevented.
- **Allergens:** An allergen is a substance which can cause an allergic reaction. What are the causes of an allergic reaction? It has been said that "Every thing under the Sun and the Sun himself can cause an allergic reaction". *The common causes are: drugs, pollen, animal dander, house-mites, dust, absorbed foods and so on.*
- **Route of contact:** Allergic reactions may occur in *various parts of the body* after exposure to different substances coming into contact with the body by different routes such as inhalation, application to the skin for topical or systemic effect, ocular conjunctiva, by nose, orally, or by parenteral route.

Ask the patient questions about: (a) Symptoms of allergy; their seasonality; (b) The possible contact with an allergen, particularly a drug or a food, if known; (c) The possible route of contact, oral (drug or food), (d) Local application (drug, cosmetics, deodorants; (d) Inhaled dust or pollen as described above); and (e) Family history of allergy.

Travel and Stay in Other Parts of the Country or Abroad

Travelling exposes a person to various infections and infestations (G.I. infections, malaria, filariasis, Hepatitis A, H.I.V., other virus infections, tuberculosis, leishmaniasis, guinea worms and other worms); injuries and so on. These may be the result of visiting an area which is known to be endemic for that particular infection; visiting such places should be avoided. Infections and infestations may be: water and food borne fecal-orally transmitted substances, air borne (tuberculosis, chemicals or insect borne (malaria, filariasis).

Did you follow the recommended precautions, e. g. the precautions against water borne and food borne infections, which are summarized as 'boil it, cook it, peel it or leave it'; Immunizations? (yellow fever, typhoid, cholera, hepatitis A); Did you take prophylactic anti-malarial drugs and other measures to avoid getting malaria? Any illness while traveling? What were the symptoms? What treatment was taken? What was the response?

Or did the illness start after returning home? Any illness which begins soon after returning home from such a visit-out should arouse the suspicion of a travel-related illness.

History of drug ingestion: Chapter 10

Information from hospitals and other doctors, and social worker's report: **Chapter 9.**

Chapter 18

Physical Examination (P.E.), Introduction

One finger in the throat and one in the rectum (of a child, my words) make a good diagnostician (William Osler).

We have learnt in Chapter 7 what Physical Examination (P. E.) means. It is the ritual of the part by part, bedside (clinical) examination, by a doctor, of a patient's body, to detect/confirm an abnormality in any part of the body and to establish what is normal in him. (Everything else is history). This contrasts with the physician and the medical students sitting in the side-room, viewing and discussing the patient's data stored in a computer (the data being called an 'i-patient'); whereas the patient rests in the ward and is called an 'icon' of the i-patient. (Culture Shock by Abraham Verghese).

Touching the patient is an important part of the P.E.. It has great therapeutic value as it establishes a bond of confidence between the doctor and the patient. (Abraham Verghese, Chapter 8).

The basic principles of History Taking remain relatively the same for all organs and organ systems in the body. The Physical Examination may differ from organ to organ and organ system to organ system. For example, the steps of physical examination will be different in the heart, the C.N.S., the ear-nose and throat, the pelvic organs, the bones and joints, and the skin.

The P.E. is broadly divided into clinical techniques such as (1) Observation = Inspection including that of the skin + non-verbal communication + minimal palpation; (2) **P**alpation; (3) **P**ercussion; and (4) **A**uscultation. The related acronym is **I.P.P.A.** The other common clinical techniques are: C.N.S.

examination; smell, hearing; rectal and vaginal examinations; trans-illumination; succussion splash; otoscopy; direct vision fundoscopy.

- Examples of inspection (a non-technique-dependent procedure) are visual recognition of emaciation, anemia, jaundice, clubbing, cutaneous striae, edema and non-verbal communication (Chapter 22).
- Examples of technique-dependent procedures are examination of the lungs, heart, abdomen and central nervous system.
- Specialties such as pediatrics, ophthalmology, orthopedics, gynecology, etc. have their own techniques to be followed.

Definitions of some techniques of physical examination:

(1) **Observation:** see above.

(2) **Inspection** is having a trained, close look at the different parts of the patient's body; their position; and their movements or lack of them.

(3) **Palpation** Chapter 19.

(4) **Percussion** is striking a finger of one hand **(Pleximeter finger)**, laid flat and firmly on the organ to be percussed with the tip of the middle finger **(Plexor aka Plessor finger)** of the opposite hand. The purpose of percussion is to: (a) Elicit resonance and dullness—lungs, abdomen; (b) Delineate the borders of the heart and the liver; palpation has now largely replaced percussion to define the heart borders (Bates); and (c) Decide whether a solid left sided abdominal lump is the splenic or renal.

Thump gently with a fist on the spine and the right lobe of the liver to elicit tenderness.

(5) **Auscultation** is listening, *with a stethoscope*, to the lungs (for breath sounds, adventitious sounds-rhonchi and rales); heart (for heart sounds and murmurs); abdomen (for peristaltic sounds, bruits and fetal heart sounds); arteries and the skull for a bruit (murmur).

For sounds generated in the patient's body, and audible (a) With the naked ears at the bedside; or (b) Through the stethoscope, which has been just lifted completely from contact with the chest wall, see Chapter 22.

The P.E. generally follows the head-to-toe sequence. The findings of observation in normal persons are called **Physical Findings**, including their normal variations (Chapters 3, 4); and the abnormalities found on P. E. in a patient are called the **Physical Signs.**

One may deviate from the **head-to-toe sequence** if it is appropriate. For example, if a suspicious or definite abnormality is detected anywhere during the head-to-toe examination, one should halt the further sequential examination, and concentrate on the abnormality and all related bodily structures and organs. For example, if you think there might be or there is (a) a Goiter, then concentrate on it: pulse, the thyroid, the trachea, the draining lymph nodes, and the eyes; (b) a lymph node, then concentrate on the area of drainage of the lymph node, all other lymph nodes in the body, and the spleen; or (c) a palpable thrill, then concentrate on the arterial structures up-stream and down-stream to the thrill, including the heart. Then, return to the head-to-toe sequential examination.

If a lesion such as an easily visible goiter or any other lump is obvious before starting the sequential P.E., examine the lesion and related structures/organs first, and then start the head-to-toe examination.

Chapter 19

Physical Examination, Principles

Symptoms are the body's mother tongue; signs are in a foreign language (Anonymous).

The physical Examination (P.E.) is carried out under the following heads:

(1) **General examination:** Observation = Inspection including that of the skin + minimal palpation if required; Nonverbal communication; Hearing and Smell.

(2) **Regional examinations:** Head and scalp; eyes; ears; nose; mouth; teeth; tongue and throat; neck which includes lower jaw; thyroid; arterial and venous pulsations; lymph nodes; axillae; breasts; liver; spleen; kidneys; groins and genitals; upper and lower limbs.

The regional examinations may have their own techniques.

(3) **Systemic examination:** R.S., C.V.S. (**I**nspection, **P**alpation, **P**ercussion and **A**uscultation; Abdomen (**I**nspection, **A**uscultation, **P**ercussion and **P**alpation).

(4) C.N.S. examination which does not follow the I.P.P.A. protocol. It has its own protocol.

The normal findings in many of the regions in the body are given in Chapter 4.

Inspection (Trained visual examination) of the patient begins as soon as you set your eyes on him and lasts as long as he is in your presence. You may be examining him in your *own clinic, the O.P.D or the ward of a hospital, at his home; or on the road* (injured or unconscious), *where you have to examine him 'as is, where is'.* You have a choice in the first four situations; on the road, you have no choice.

- **Preparation of the examination area in the first four sites.** It should be clean, well lit and quiet. On the road, it is 'as is, where is'.
- The **Lighting** may be:
- **Diffuse** light (daylight and fluorescent-tube light) reflected by the walls and the ceiling is fine for most purposes.
- **Strong** light from a hand-held shadow-less flashlight is generally preferred for procedures such as a puncture or a biopsy.
- **Strong, tangential** (oblique) light from a pen-torch, held at a slight angle close to the surface to be examined, shows up better the irregularities of the surface such as small elevations and depressions; just visible goiter; and any movement under the skin (jugular venous pulsations and pressure and cardiac apex impulse) and the abdominal wall (visible intestinal peristalses).
- **Strong light** from a pen torch with a good reflector in it is necessary for examination of the mouth and throat. In a darkened room, it is used for testing pupillary reactions and trans-illumination; the last test is a poor test and has low Diagnostic Accuracy (see Chapter 20).
- **Preparation of the patient:** Make certain that the patient is sitting or lying down comfortably. Avoid making a weak or seriously ill patient change his position often.

- **Chaperone:** If you are examining a female patient, then a nurse, a lady relative or a female attendant should be standing by the side of the patient, to give her a sense of security, especially if you are going to examine the patient's chest, abdomen or genitals. Such a person is called a chaperone.
- **Patient's position:** see later
- **Physician's position:** Stand or sit on the right side of the patient and use your right hand for examination. Bend down or sit at the patient's level for examination of the abdomen.
- **Explanation:** Explain to the patient what you are going to do, especially if the examination is going to be painful or embarrassing.
- **Exposure:** Make the patient expose only the part of the body which you are going to examine; after the examination is over, cover up the exposed part.

Palpation is examination by touching the different parts of the patient's body with the examiner's hand. There is hardly an accessible part of the body that is not amenable to palpation. Palpation may be (a) Uni-manual, light (in the case of abdomen, not depressing the palpated surface more than 1cm, Mosby's book), medium or deep, for examination of the abdomen and other organs and structures in the body; (b) One hand on the top of the other for deep abdominal palpation; and (c) Bimanual (using both hands) for palpation of the Liver, Spleen and Kidneys (patient supine); Breasts (patient upright); Uterus and Adnexae (patient in **dorsal recumbent position** = supine + lower limbs bent and soles of the feet touching the bed; **recumbent** = lying down). (d) **Palpation of the Precordium:** Palpation has now replaced Precordial Percussion for determining the size of the heart.

Optimum use of your hands for palpation: Use

The ball of the hand (the bony part of the palm at the base of the fingers) or **the ulnar border of hand** for feeling transmitted vibration such as the tactile fremitus in chest examination.

Dorsal surface of hand or fingers: for estimating body temperature.

Palmar Surface of the middle three (2nd to 4th) fingers and their underlying finger pads (soft tissue): for Position, Shape, Size, Texture, Consistency, Tenderness, Mobility and shape of a lump, and other attributes of lesions such as Fluid and Crepitus. The breast is best palpated with palmer surfaces of the middle three (2nd, 3rd and 4th) fingers and their finger pads (*called palpation by the flat of the hand*) for detecting and confirming a round and soft lump (*fibroadenoma or cyst*), or a irregularly shaped, hard mass (*cancer*).

Palpation is also valuable for examining *arteries*, cardiac and arterial *thrills*, precordial area, *joints* and *bones*; *eyeballs*; and for *rectal* and *vaginal* examination.

Patient's Position During Physical Examination

Much of the physical examination can be carried out with the patient either lying supine in the bed, or sitting on a stool, as per local custom and convenience. **Supine** position = lying on the back with arms by the sides and legs extended, for examining the thorax, lungs, heart and abdomen; groins and lower limbs.

Some of the other positions are:

- **Patient sitting in a chair, with back supported, or lying down comfortably**, for five minutes before measurement of blood pressure (Hutchison's book).
- **Patient sitting up for specialist examination** of eyes, ears, nose, mouth, teeth and throat.

- **Dorsal recumbent position** for examination of breasts, axillae, front and sides of lungs, heart, abdomen, groins, female external genitals, the lower limbs.
- With the **patient supine, the head of the bed raised 30 degrees** for jugular venous pulse pressure and pulsations.
- **Supine patient rolled over partly to the left side or fully to the left lateral recumbent position** for auscultation of the heart, especially the low pitched, diastolic murmur of mitral stenosis.
- Patient **sitting, bent forwards** and exhaling, for the high pitched diastolic murmur of aortic regurgitation.
- **Supine, left and right lateral recumbent positions (one after the another)** for testing for ascites (except when a small amount of fluid is present, which requires ultrasonography to be done).
- **Lying supine, then sitting, and finally standing** for testing for postural hypotension.
- **Right lateral recumbent position** for palpation of a difficult-to-palpate spleen (Mosby).
- **Left lateral recumbent position** with the right knee and hip flexed sharply, and the bottom leg flexed slightly (Sim's position) for rectal examination.
- **Physician standing behind the patient sitting on a stool** for examining the thyroid, posterior lungs and back of the thorax and of the neck.
- **Do not auscultate the back of the lungs in either left or right lateral recumbent position** because the greater ventilation in the dependent lung can lead to false asymmetry in physical signs between the two lungs (Bates). Auscultate the back of the lungs with the patient sitting.

- The **female patient lying supine in the bed, sitting up or standing** for breast examination, including the bimanual examination.
- **Standing** male patient for examination of the external genitals.
- **Lithotomy position:** Female patient in dorsal recumbent position (see above), buttocks brought down to the lower edge of the table for external gynecological examination; plus legs in stirrups for internal gynecological examination.
- **Positions for** rectal examination: See GI system in Chapter 28.
- **Prone** position (lying on the stomach) for specialized orthopedic tests such as 'knee flexion test' and 'hip rotation test'.

Compare

Compare an abnormality in any part of the body (a) With the same in the corresponding part on the opposite side, whenever possible; (b) With what you have Seen, Measured and Recorded in the past; and (c) With the help of Published Tables, with persons of similar age (contemporaries), same gender and same race.

It is advisable to **examine all the normal, unaffected systems as well in each patient, even if the diagnosis is obvious.** This alone will give you an idea of what the normal abdomen feels like, what the normal heart sounds/murmurs and breath sounds are like, what the normal knee jerk and plantar reflex are like and so on. This will help you to recognize the abnormal physical signs with confidence.

Valuation of Physical Signs (see Chapter 20).

Health Precautions

Washing hands: Wash your hands with soap and water, or scrub them with a lotion (Sterillium), containing alcohol + an antiseptic, before and after the P.E. of each patient, in order to prevent transmission of infection.

Wear gloves in some cases; remember that latex can cause a local allergic reaction.

If H.I.V. in on the cards, remember that there is **no** tissue/ secretion/excretion in the body which has **never** transmitted H.I.V.. A handshake is generally safe if the skin is not abraded or cut.

Some Commonly Used Simple Gadgets

- **Stethoscope:** The stethoscope should have a double chest-piece, a **diaphragm** (for high-pitched sounds such as an aortic diastolic murmur); and a shallow **bell** with a large diameter (for low-pitched sounds such as a mitral diastolic murmur, the Korotkoff sounds during blood press measurement, bowel sounds and the arterial bruit in the abdomen). The **ear pieces** should fit your ears snugly and comfortably. The bell should be applied to the chest wall and the arm lightly for this purpose. If you press the bell on the skin, the skin becomes taut, and acts like a diaphragm. The stethoscope should be from 12 inches to not more than 18 inches in **length**. The **tubing** should be thick and heavy for good conduction of sound.
- **Pen torch:** It should provide a strong central beam of light for examining the tongue and throat, testing pupillary reactions, and, in a darkened room, for testing trans-illumination of the paranasal sinuses

(for pus), scrotum (for hydrocele) and adult female breasts (for a lesion and bleeding). However, transillumination has low **diagnostic accuracy** (D. A; see chapter 20). The pen torch is also used as source of a tangential beam of light when required (see above).

- **Tuning forks:** There should be a tuning fork with frequency about 128 cps for testing vibration sense; and another one with frequency either 256 cps or 512 cps for testing hearing.
- **Tendon hammer** for eliciting tendon reflexes.

Chapter 20

Valuation of Physical Signs

Erroneous assumptions can be disastrous (Peter F. Drucker).

Clinicians have been using physical signs for over 100 years for examining the patients. Some physical signs are strong indicators of the presence or absence of a disease condition (i. e. they have **High Diagnostic Accuracy**, D.A.) and therefore are very helpful diagnostically. Others are weak indicators (i. e, **Low Diagnostic Accuracy**, D.A.) and, therefore, are not helpful. The following table by John M. Naish was one attempt to divide the physical signs clinically into very helpful, somewhat helpful and unhelpful in clinical practice.

Since the 1940s, powerful diagnostic techniques (ultrasonography, C.T. scan and M.R.I. scan) have become available. They can detect even small differences in the shape, size or functioning (M.R.I.) of some internal organs with high resolution and accuracy.

It is *erroneous* to assume that all physical signs are equally efficient diagnostically. The *disaster* is consequences of wrong diagnosis. Scientists thought that the time had come to compare old traditional physical signs with their modern instrumental counterparts, and determine how well the signs performed compared with the new Gold Standard tests in ruling in or ruling out the disease condition they are expected to detect or rule out, i.e. their D. A., in a given clinical setting, in a *defined population* e. g. men vs women; the young vs the elderly; in general practice vs specialty practice.

The valuation can be done either by **collective clinical experience and its critical analysis** (see Naish's table); or **mathematically (Evidence Based Physical Diagnosis)**. The latter is a complicated but generally a more efficient procedure.

Collective experience of the correct use of physical signs:

- Everybody, everywhere, must perform technique-dependent tests (see Chapter 7) in identical manner; this is difficult. However, the availability of DVDs and iPads containing videos of some of the technique-dependent tests (Chapter 7) is helpful in this matter.
- Collective clinical experience suggests the following points:

1. A qualitative test, e.g. plantar reflex, which gives a yes/no answer has a higher D. A. than an ordinal (graded) test e.g. muscle strength, knee jerk or a systolic heart murmur. Diastolic cardiac murmurs (mitral and aortic) have higher D. A. than systolic murmurs. A pansystolic mumur of tricuspid regurgitation has very high D. A. (see below).
2. A test with narrow normal range e. g. body temperature has higher D. A. than one with a wide range of normal, say pulse rate (see table below).
3. With bilaterally symmetrical body systems, asymmetry in the physical signs between the two sides e. g. diminished or increased intensity of breath sounds or dullness on percussion has a high D. A. On the other hand, bilaterally depressed ankle jerks in the elderly may be a normal variant. Beware of the asymmetry of the thoracic organs in the symmetrical thoracic cage (see Chapter 26).
4. The variation in the innate ability for resolution possessed by the different human sense organs employed to elicit a physical sign has a major influence. **Measurement, the use of eyes, touch, hearing and smell stand in a diminishing order of ability** to differentiate between the normal and the abnormal (see table below).
5. Intra- and inter-observer variation i.e. disagreement among observers in their detecting the various

abnormalities, is an important cause of diagnostic difficulty.

6. Awareness of the age-wise and gender-wise differences in pulse rate and blood pressure, those in special circumstances such as pregnancy (Chapter 6) and ethnic differences in the skin, hair and oral mucosal appearance is important in not falling into the trap of diagnosing a non-existent disease e. g. diagnosis Addison's disease from dark oral mucosal patches in the Dravidian population of south India.
7. Negative signs may be of critical importance in making a diagnosis, and may have a high D.A. e. g. the absence of elevated jugular venous pressure in a person with hepatic enlargement makes congestive heart failure an unlikely cause of the enlarged liver.
8. Most physical signs increase or decrease the probability of a given disease process being present, but they may not be absolutely (100%) diagnostic. When we label a physical sign as 'diagnostic' of something, we should be actually saying that it is 'highly suggestive', at least in most instances.
9. But, a left lower parasternal, pan-systolic murmur is 100% accurate and diagnostic; it has very high D. A. in the diagnosis of tricuspid regurgitation (Stephen McGee).

Similarly, it is very difficult to diagnose small quantities of fluid in the peritoneal cavity with the old, obsolete clinical technique of percussion. But, sometimes it may be the only method available for that purpose because of non availability of the gold standard method viz ultrasonography. Similarly, transillumination is a poor test with low D.A.

Evidence-based physical diagnosis is a part of Evidence-Based Medicine (E.B.M.)

It is a sophisticated numerical expression (quantification) of what a physician does mentally when examining a patient. A tremendous amount of spade-work by medical scientists has gone into building the data bases required for the purpose.

From the history given by the patient, the examining physician prepares mentally a list of possible diagnoses (differential diagnosis). While examining the patient, he constantly adds to or deletes from the initial list of possible diagnoses. He does this by considering his experience of the importance or otherwise of every physical sign that he elicits, and then modifies and perhaps narrows the differential diagnosis. He keeps on saying to himself "Sign A is present/absent and this increases the possibility of disease X; or Sign B is present/absent and that decreases the possibility of disease Y".

The terms used in E.B.M., Two by two table, Sensitivity, Specificity, Intra- and inter-observer variation, True positive, True negative, False positive, False negative, Positive/Negative Predictability, Pre-and Post-test Probability and 'Likelihood Ratio' (L.R.) are not easy to master.

In simple words, sensitivity means assurance that if something is expected to be found, it will be found. Similarly, specificity means assurance that if something is found, it will be a true finding.

Let us look at two terms from the above list: **Pre-test probability and Likelihood ratio.**

Pre-test probability of a disease in a patient is equal to its prevalence in the population of which he is a member. The clinician can find out from the literature an estimate of such prevalence and hence of the pre-test probability of the condition under consideration.

He will also be able to find out from the literature another number termed **Likelihood ratio (L.R.)** which tells us whether and how much a given physical sign increases or decreases the pre-test probability of the disease under consideration. For example, a given physical sign increases the pre-test probability of the disease by 40%. This information alone is not sufficient in making a diagnosis unless the pre-test probability is also known. If the pre-test probability is 50% (the disease is common in the population) and the L. R. increases it by 40%, the post-test probability is 50% + 40 % = 90%, with high D.A. If the disease has a pre-test probability of 1% (the disease is rare in the population), the post-test probability, using the same physical sign, is 1% + 40% = 41%, and the D.A. of the same physical sign is low.

The prevalence of a disease varies with composition of the population the patient comes from e.g. a General practitioner's clinic, an Internal medicine specialist's patients or a Cardiologist's patients; further the setting in which the patient is being seen (as an acute emergency case or as a cold case), and the patient's general health, co-morbidities and so on. Therefore, L.R. has to be adjusted by each clinician in each patient according to the information from his own practice. That requires access to a computer for storing the data and for calculations while going around in the ward from patient to patient. *This is not easy for a practicing clinician in his busy daily practice, and for the over-burdened students.*

Some clinicians and medical teachers have reservations about teaching E.B.M. to students. However, a clinician's mind works along the same lines as E. B. M. during an evaluation of a patient. He keeps on saying to himself "This finding is present and makes it more likely that disease A rather than disease B is present ".

To be universally useful, dedicated databases such as those of pretest probability and L.R. will have to be updated periodically. Perhaps, it will then be a matter of opportune time, availability of low-cost and capable, smartphones and phablets, and easy access to the mother data bases, that Evidence Based Physical Diagnosis will become routine in clinical teaching and daily clinical practice.

Clinical Valuation of Physical Signs

Sense mainly employed	Wide variation of normal	Narrow variation of normal	Value of physical sign
Measurement (All senses and time)	Pulse rate		B
		Temperature	A
	Blood pressure		B
Eyes	Size of the abdomen		C
		Raised jugular venous pressure	A
	Facial, axillary and pubic hair		E
	Muddy sclera		C
		Jaundice	B
Touch	Liver edge just palpable		D
		Spleen palpable	A
Hearing	Impaired vocal resonance		E
		Aortic diastolic murmur	A
	Quality of voice		E
Smell	Offensive breath		F
		Smell of anaerobic infection	B

A represents the highest diagnostic rating, and F the lowest. Modified from Clinical Apprentice by John M. Naish. and Alfred A.E. Read., Published by John Wright & Sons, Bristol, 1978.

Chapter 21

Measurement in Medicine

When you can measure what you are speaking about, and express it in numbers, you know something about it; when you cannot express it in numbers, your knowledge is of a meager and unsatisfactory kind (Lord Kelvin).

Measurement has an important place in clinical medicine. It comprises (1), **M**easurement; (2) **C**ounting; (3) **R**atios; and (4) **D**ifference (MCRD). Repeated MCRD are more informative than a single measurement.

Primary Measurements

Measurement: The generally measured parameters in adults are: (a) Body temperature; (b) Blood pressure; (c) Standing height; (d) Upper segment of the body = US.; (e) Lower segment of the body (LS); (f) Body weight; (g) Arm span; (h) Chest circumference; (i) Chest expansion; (j) Abdominal girth; (k) Waist circumference and (l) Hip circumference.

Counting: The two countable attributes are (a) Pulse rate; and (b) Respiratory rate.

Temperature, pulse rate, respiratory rate (T, P, R) and blood pressure grouped together are known as the **Vital Signs** (see Chapter 23).

Derived Measurements

Ratio and difference: The important ratios in adults are:

(a) Waist/Hip (circumference) ratio; (i) US/LS ratio and (ii) Body Mass Index which is an index percentage of body fat (see Chapter 23) and acts as indicator of overweight, obesity, normal weight and underweight;

(b) Ankle Brachial Index assesses the adequacy of arterial circulation in the feet at the bedside (Stanford Medicine 25 on the internet gives details).

(c) Normal Arm Span is longer than the standing height by up to 5 cm. ***A larger difference together with a U/L ratio less than 1.0/1.0*** (eunuchoidal proportions) in adult men and women suggest hypogonadism of prepubertal onset.

Lord Kelvin's statement about what can be measured and expressed in numbers and what cannot be (see above) is famous. Clinical medicine provides an exception to the second half of Kelvin's statement. Much good clinical medicine can be practised in the absence of facilities to measure. An example is the experienced clinicians noticing intuitively a small change in a seriously ill patient's condition, and deciding whether he is improving or deteriorating, even when the tests are not available or they turn out to be unhelpful. Therefore, well developed **clinical acumen** sometimes proves to be superior to physical/ chemical measurements.

Chapter 22

General Examination, Introduction

There is no more difficult art to acquire than the art of observation (Osler).

General examination of the patient begins as soon as you first look at the him and lasts as long as the he is in your presence. It covers the general assessment of the health and the personality of the patient primarily by **OBSERVATION** (= Trained inspection + minimal palpation if required); **LOOK; SMELL; HEAR; THINK-AND-GUESS**. The patient is touched only when necessary.

It does not include the systemic examinations (R.S., C.V.S., G.I. and C.N.S.) and the regional examinations (thyroid, liver, spleen and so on).

In this and subsequent chapters on physical examination, an attempt has been made to provide 'Normal Physical Findings' in different parts of the body, if they are not provided in Chapter 4. Chapter 4 and each the following chapters should be read together.

Look (Inspection = look closely)

- Look over the patient **from head to toe** with minimal touching, without examining any part in detail and without disrobing him. Does he look apparently healthy or unwell?
- **Is the mental state normal?** Does he recognize you? Talks and listens well? Takes interest in surroundings? Is he alert; well orientated; or drowsy; delirious; or comatose?

- **Stature and build.** Stature is height. Build is difficult to express in numbers.
- **Does he look well nourished?**
- **Evidence of malnutrition?** (a) **Weight loss** (redundant skin in rapid weight loss); Fatiguability; Cold intolerance; Pallor; signs of Vitamin Deficiency such as Glossitis; Stomatitis; Koilonychia; Xerophthalmia; Skin pigmentation; Dermatitis; Ankle edema; and (b) The state of the **skeletal muscles.**
- The Nutritional State is recorded as either 'well nourished' or 'poorly nourished'.
- **Signs of dehydration?** Diminished Elasticity and Turgor of the skin; excessive Thirst, and the Dry appearance and feel of the oral mucosa.
- **Gait:** How he walks, at what speed, uses any assistive devices?
- **Posture:** What position he maintains continuously while, standing, sitting, lying down.
- **Movement:** How he **gets up** from the chair or from bed?
- **Face** appears Happy, Sullen, Aggressive, Cooperative, Uncooperative, Indifferent?
- **Comfortable** or in pain, breathless or emotionally distressed? (see Chapter 23 for definition).
- **Tidy or shabby** including tobacco-stained fingers?
- **Well dressed**, appropriately for age. **Well groomed** = taking good care of nails, teeth, hair, skin, clean shaven, beard, if present; uses spectacles?
- **Does he look you** in the eye? Or avoids your gaze?
- **Gross asymmetry** in bilateral organs?

- **Do his hearing and eyesight appear normal?**
- Is **he obese? Obvious weight loss?**
- **Skin** as much as you can see without disrobing the patient.
- **Gross, visible evidence of a disease?** A Swelling, Lump; Bleeding; Ulceration or loss of tissue anywhere; Facial flush; Thumping arterial pulse in the neck; Pallor (anemia); Shortness of breath; Cyanosis; Jaundice; Edema (feet, face, elsewhere); Deformity; Paresis; Paralysis; Involuntary Movements such as tics, tremor, head nodding; mannerisms, and more.
- **An injury which can occur, or a wound which is inflicted?**

Smell

Can you appreciate **around the patient** any foul or unnatural odour such as occurs in recent Alcohol consumption, Diabetic coma, Anaerobic infection, Atrophic rhinitis, Uremia, Pulmonary suppuration and Pyorrhea?

Hear at the bedside:

(a) Can you hear **at the bedside** any abnormal sound such as Coughing; Groaning; Wheezing; Borborygmi, Stertor, or Stridor coming from the patient, or (change in) patient's voice e.g. Hoarseness or Feeble voice?

Stertor: This is low pitched (like snoring), noisy breathing, always inspiratory, *due to obstruction above larynx.* Cyanosis and tracheal tug may be present. It is commoner in children than in adults (Dr. Balu).

Stridor: It is low-to-high pitched, noisy breathing, both inspiratory and expiratory, and may be musical. It is accompanied by cough, hoarseness, dyspnoea, and choking. It is due to an obstruction in the *larynx, trachea or bronchi* (Balu).

It is difficult to learn to recognize some of these sounds merely by reading a book or hearing a lecture. If you are in the ward long enough to hear these sounds emanating from a patient, you might be able to recognize them the next time you hear them. Take-home message: **Spend as much time in the ward as you can**. "It [the ward] is your temple of learning; and the patients are gods" (Anonymous).

(b) A grade-6 cardiac murmur, accompanied by a thrill, where the palpable murmur, is so loud that it continues to be audible even after the chest piece is just removed from contact with the chest wall.

Think-and-Guess

Nonverbal (silent, speechless) communication occurs continuously between any two or more persons sitting together. It is reading the body language which is based on observing the posture (Nadkarni), and other physical activities of a person: (a) how he walks, stands, sits or lies down; and (b) other non-verbal signals such as facial expression, looking in the eye, smiling, growling, tics such as clenching the fist, and so on. These observations permit the observer to guess the mental makeup, attitude, feelings and emotions of, say, a patient or an interviewee. All the observations should be interpreted in the context of the individual's cultural background.

Chapter 23

General Examination, Continued

One swallow does not a summer make, but one tophus makes gout and one crescent, malaria (Willium Osler).

Measure whatever you can, and record it. If it is not found in the record later, you have not carried out the examination in the first instance. Even a crude measurement is better than a vague description such as apple sized, pea sized, egg sized and so on.

Vital Signs

The vital signs have been defined as: 'Results of tests used to gauge whether a patient's physiological systems are functioning sufficiently well to support survival and provide a platform for achieving wellness.'

The **conventional** vital signs used in adults are:

(1) Temperature: Normal oral temperature varies during the day. It is lower in the early hours of morning (as low 35.80-C) and higher in the late evening (as high 37.70C; Circadian rhythm). Oral temperature of more than 37.80C is fever. Remember that the oral temperature is raised by sustained smoking and chewing for 20 minutes.

(2) Pulse rate: Normal rate is 50-95/minute Rate less than 50 is bradycardia, and more than 100 is tachycardia.

(3) Respiratory rate: Count it without letting the patient being aware that you are counting his breaths. Normal respiratory rate is variously quoted as from (12-18) breaths per minute to (16-25) breaths per minute (McGee).

(4) Blood pressure: *"The blood pressure is measured with the patient sitting. Measure it with the arm at the heart level, after the patient has been sitting quietly in a chair with back supported, for at least five minutes"*; this is the standard recommendation. If the patient is too weak to sit up, it may be measured in the supine position. Use the bell as the Korotkoff sounds are low pitched. The recommendation of sitting up is based on the consensus of opinion of the expert committees who reviewed all the scientific data (McGee). *However, the exact reason for this preference for the sitting posture is not stated explicitly anywhere.* For stethoscope, see Chapter 19.

Record the position of the patient and the side of the arm in which B.P. was measured, along with the figures of systolic and diastolic blood pressure. On all future occasions, measure the blood pressure in the same arm and in the same patient position as the first time. At the first patient visit, measure the B.P. in both arms. Normal blood pressure in the arm, during resting, is 100/60 to 120/80.

A difference of more than 10 mm Hg systolic B.P. between two arms suggests the possibility of a proximal arterial block. Normally, the femoral pulse is palpable before the simultaneous radial pulse; in coarctation of the aorta, the reverse is true (radio-femoral delay).

Some new vital signs:

(5) Pain: Severe, unbearable and not responding to treatment.

(6) Emotional distress which is extreme discomfort because of pain, dyspnoea, financial worry, guilt, anxiety due to fear or uncertainty about the future in seriously/terminally ill patients, commonly those with cancer.

(7) The six minutes walking test to assess cardio-respiratory functional status in the elderly, especially preoperatively.

Other Measurements

Height: A recent publication on this topic is 'Secular Trends in Height in India' by Mamidi R.S. et. al. 'Pooled data from 65245 men and 118796 women (age 20-49 years) from 29 states analyzed; Food and Nutrition Bulletin; 32:1, 2011 (Sponsor: United Nations University).

The ***average height*** of Indian men was 165 cm, and that of Indian women was 152 cm. in that study. These were *'all-India' figures. State-wise,* the average height was the highest (168.4 cm in men and 157.5 cm in women) in the Jammu-Kashmir, a northern state, and the lowest (154.7 cm in men and 149.3 cm in women) in *Meghalaya., a north-eastern state. In Maharashtra, a Western state, it was 165.7 cm in men and 152.3 cm in women.*

Body weight and body mass index: To be clinically meaningful, body weight must be interpreted in terms of the height. This is done by calculating Body Mass Index (B.M.I.). The latter is an estimate of the patient' *percent body fat mass.* There is a curvilinear relation between B.M.I. and *percent body fat mass.* However, *the current practical definition of obesity is based on the relationship between B.M.I. and health outcome rather than on B.M.I. and body* composition. (Williams Endocrinology, Edition 12, Chapter 36)

Body Mass Index is calculated as: B.M.I. = Weight (kg)/ Height2 (meter).

B.M.I. < 18.5 means underweight; 18.5-24.9 is normal; 25.00-29.9 means overweight; 30.00-39.9 means obesity; and 40.00 and higher levels mean extreme obesity.

B.M.I. less than 18.5 is a risk factor (increased future probability) for diseases due to being underweight.

B.M.I. of 25.00 and higher is a risk factor for diabetes mellitus, hypertension, cardiovascular disease and stroke. In Asian-Indians, this cut-off figure for determining the risk factor is 23.00.

The B.M.I. has two limitations (a) It does not tell you whether the elevated body weight is due to excess fat or due to well developed muscles which are heavier than fat; and (b) It does not tell you whether the fat accumulation is upper abdominal i.e. visceral, which occurs is in men, or in thighs and buttocks which occurs in women. The accumulation of visceral fat predicts increased future probability of diabetes and related conditions (see above); lower body accumulation of fat i. e. in thighs and buttocks, does not so predict unless the accumulation is massive.

Waist/Hip ratio=Measure of Central Obesity. It is inconvenient to measure the waist circumference.

Waist circumference is probably the best solution to these problems at present. It is easier to measure than hip circumference which is required for calculating waist/hip ratio If waist circumference is 102.00 cm or higher in men and 88.00 cm or higher in women; it is considered to be a risk factor for the conditions mentioned above, irrespective of the B.M.I.

Chapter 24

Head and Neck

A good head and a good heart are always a formidable combination (Nelson Mandela).

After the general examination comes the examination of organ systems (R.S., C.V.S., G.I.S., and C.N.S.); and the regional examinations. The total physical examination is carried out in an head to toe sequence: (1) Head and Neck; (2) Skin and its appendages, Breasts, Axillae and Upper limbs; (3) Thorax- this includes the Thoracic cage, Respiratory system (R.S.) and Cardiovascular System (C.V.S.); (5) Abdomen; (6) Groins, External genitals and lower limbs; and (7) Central Nervous system.

What follows in this and subsequent chapters is what abnormalities to look for in different sites in the body during physical examination. The technique of examination is generally not described; the interpretation often is.

Head and Associated Structures

Head

Normal: Shape oval and symmetrical; size measured as circumference about 56 cm (22"); surface may be lumpy.

General observations: History of boxing and contact sports; Abnormal shape such as microcephly and possibly Mental retardation.

Examine for size too large (hydrocephalus) or too small (generalized craniostenosis); *abnormal shape* (asymmetry, scapocephaly, dolicocephaly, brachycephaly); *lump; depression; deformit; tenderness, involuntary movement* (Paralysis agitans).

Face: (Face is the mirror to health).

Normal: See Chapter 4. Scanty facial hair in men may be a racial normal variant. Chloasma in parous women is normal. Positive Chvostek's sign is rarely a normal variant.

Examine for ageing lines around the mouth; Dark pigmentation (consider Addison's disease); Rounded moon face (Cushing's syndrome); Absence of facial expression (mask face of Parkinsonism); Facial asymmetry; Facial nerve paralysis; Facial tics; Acne; Hirsutism; Oily face in women and children (consider administration or excess production of androgen as the cause—commonest cause in women is *polycystic ovary* syndrome; in children therapeutic androgen (*anabolic steroids administration*); *congenital adrenal hyperplasia.* Scanty facial hair in men—may be a normal variant, but think of hypogonadism; Loss of outer ⅓rd of eyebrows (hypothyroidism); Puffiness or edema (hypothyroidism, kidney disease, on waking in the morning in congestive heart failure; superior mediastinal syndrome); *learn to recognize* some typical appearances of the face such as acromegalic, cretinoid, hyperthyroid, infantile, Mongoloid, Hippocratic and more; Twitching of upper lip on tapping the facial nerve in front of the pinna (Chvostek's sign of hypocalcemia); Tenderness of the superficial temporal artery in front of the pinna (giant cell arteritis) which can lead to severe headache and even blindness; Palpable parotid salivary gland? It is not palpable in health; tenderness (parotitis, mumps), enlargement (parotitis, duct obstruction, tumour). Submandibular salivary glands—similar to parotid glands. Palpate the temporomandibular joints while the patient opens and closes mouth.

External eyes: Before starting the examination, think of Vision; Field of vision; Fundoscopy in diagnosis in internal medicine. Mongoloid race; mongolism (Down syndrome).

Normal: See Chapter 4. A tiny difference between the size of the two pupils, not appreciated by naked eye, is a normal variant, if the papillary reactions are normal. Horizontal diplopia may be physiologic under certain circumstances. A few beats of nystagmus on the extreme lateral gaze are a normal variant. Muddy, buff coloured sclera seen in the palpebral fissure is a normal variant, not jaundice.

Examine for: Position of eyelids; Lid lag, Lid retraction and Lid drooping; Edema of eyelids; Symmetry of lines of gaze between the two eyes; Pallor and cyanosis of palpebral conjunctiva; Yellow coloration of sclera (jaundice); Kayser Fleischer rings (Wilson's disease)—seen better and earlier by slit lamp examination; Approximate acuity of vision—hand-held chart; does the patient *wear glasses*? what *kind of glasses*? Pain in and redness and tearing of the eyes; are the eyes normally *moist* or are they dry (insufficient tear production); Pupillary reaction to bright light and accomodation; Opacity in the cornea and lens; Eyeball movements in all directions.

External ears: If there is any abnormality in the ear, nose or throat (E.N.T.), examine all three.

Before starting the examination, think of Low set ear; hairy pinna only in males; congenital hairy pinna.

Normal: See Chapter 4.

Examine Pinna for Shape (normal or deformed), Size (normal or small), Position (normal; or low set as in mental retardation and syndromes such Down's syndrome, Turner syndrome). *If pain or ear discharge is present move and pull the* *pinna of the painful ear*); acuity of *hearing*—whispered voice test or ticking watch test for auditory acuity; enquire about *tinnitus* (perceived sound that has no external stimulus; compare with hallucinations); Vertigo; Locked ears; Recent air travel; examine the nose, paranasal sinuses and throat for *evidence of infection*; look into the external auditory canals and at the ear drums. Ears are called *low set* if the pinna is entirely below the line joining the outer canthus of the eye and occiput.

Nose and Paranasal Sinuses

Nose: Normal: See Chapter 4. Some asymmetry between the two nostrils is normal.

The nasal mucosa is somewhat redder than the oral mucosa; this is normal.

Examine for shape of the nose (normal—racial difference; or deformed); Evidence of recent *trauma*—fracture; Nasal *obstruction; any discharge* from the nostrils—uni- or bi-lateral; nature of discharge—Watery, Mucoid, Muco-Purulent; press on the frontal and maxillary sinuses for *tenderness*; look inside the two sides of the nose—Pallor or Edema of mucosa, Deviation of septum; Polyps; Bleeding spot; Ulceration; evidence of Nose picking (can cause nose-bleeding); Foreign body; look whether *alae nasi* are moving—if they are, it indicates that the airway resistance is markedly increased; *Smell* test—See C.N.S. Chapter; *Nose smells foul*—atrophic rhinitis.

Paranasal sinuses: finger pressure for *tenderness*—ethmoid, frontal and maxillary; Transillumination—low diagnostic accuracy (D.A.; see Chapter 20).

Mouth: See Chapter 28

Throat (pharynx)

Normal: See Chapter 4. The *tonsils* are generally small or absent in adults (normal variant). *Large* tonsils may not necessarily be abnormal but may be those that have not sufficiently regressed from childhood size. They should be carefully examined and investigated, especially if unilateral (fear of malignancy).

Examine for: Look for Colour of the oropharynx and nearby structures--tonsils, soft palate, uvula, tonsillar fossae (pink), Appearance (smooth or granular); Symmetry; Tenderness; Exudate; Swelling; Ulceration; and Tonsillar size and appearance of the surface; Midline meeting of tonsils causing *obstruction*. Ask the patient to open the mouth and say '*ah*' and carry out the above examinations. Palpate a suspicious lesion with a gloved finger. Look for a sharp object such as a fish bone *embedded* in the pharynx or a nearby structure. Note the patient's voice (hoarse, low, shrill). *Uvula* is central but a little deviation to right or left side is a normal variant.

Neck

A short neck denotes a good mind. You see, the messages go quicker to the brain because they have shorter to go (Anonymous).

The neck is the conduit (passage) between the head and the trunk, and contains the most important structures passing either way. It extends from the base of the skull above (upper limit) to the clavicles and the sternum below (lower limit). Most structures passing through the neck either way are in a closed circuit (they do not communicate with the outside atmosphere). The only exceptions are the air passage (trachea) and the food pipe (esophagus) which communicate with the outside atmosphere at their upper ends.

Normal: See Chapter 3, 4, 5 and 6. Several groups of lymph nodes (most have been given positional names) are present in the neck. They range from the harmless shotty lymph nodes in the posterior triangle to those frightening ones in the supraclavicular region (chance of metastases from the lungs or the abdomen). 'Shotty' means hard like the shots (collections) of shotgun lead pellets, small, round, discrete, mobile, and non-tender nodes which may be found in the posterior triangle in normal people. In the very crowded neck, other structures such as a small muscle or a small artery may be misdiagnosed as lymph nodes. The simple rule is that a small structure that can be rolled up and down, and side to side is a lymph node. Neither a small artery nor a bit of muscle can be rolled in this manner. An artery pulsates. A lymph node does not pulsate.

Before starting the examination, think of: Length: very short neck associated with obesity and with syndromes such as Turner syndrome and Down syndrome.

Examine for: (a) Parotid and submandibular **salivary glands** for size, a nodule and tenderness; these glands are not palpable when normal.

(b) Groups of **lymph nodes** in the neck should be palpated systematically. If any are felt, search all other neck nodes, their areas of drainage, and lymph nodes all over the body (localized versus generalized lymphadenopathy); Stress on supraclavicular infraclavicular and epitrochlear lymph nodes; if enlarged they may be harboring meastases from a thoracic or abdominal primary lesion.

(c) **Thyroid gland** (make sure that it is thyroid gland by the swallowing test); its shape, size; whether it is uniform in consistency (normal, firm or hard) or is nodular (single nodule or multinodular); Mobility; Draining lymph nodes. Do this from the front and from behind. Record these findings along with a simple diagram. Examine eyes for exophthalmos; skin for temperature; ankle jerks (normal, dull, slow and brisk); and hands for finger tremors. Auscultate the thyroid for a bruit; trachea and its position (central or pushed +/-), compressed by a mass, width, tenderness, lump; does the patient come from an iodine deficient area; history of radiation to thyroid or nearby organ.

(e) **Sternomastoid muscles**—strength, ability to turn neck, tenderness.

(f) **The internal carotid artery** *and the internal jugular vein* are in the carotid sheath which is in the anterior triangle of the neck, deep to the sternomastoid muscle. The *artery* is visible and palpable in anterior triangle. The internal jugular vein may be visible with some difficulty but not palpable. The *external jugular vein* runs downwards and backwards on the surface of the sternomastoid mucle and is more easily visible than the internal jugular vein; its terminal part dips into the posterior triangle of the neck. Measure the internal jugular vein *pressure* and study the jugular *pulsations*, in the internal jugular vein. The use of a pen torch to throw *tangential light* on the area concerned heightens the visibility of the jugular pulsations.

(g) Thickened and palpable **great auricular nerve,** obliquely crossing the sternomastoid muscle, suggests leprosy.

(h) **Webbing** of the neck and very short neck (chromosomal anomalies such as Turner syndrome).

(i) **Neck stiffness** - sprain, spinal root compression, trauma.

(j) **Neck rigidity** i.e. passive resistance to flexion of the neck in a supine patient suggests meningitis.

Chapter 25

Skin, Breasts, Axillae and Upper Limbs

Think how lucky you are that the skin you live in, so beautifully holds the "You" who's within (Michael Tyler).

Skin and its Appendages

The normal physical findings in skin, hair and nails are described in Chapter 4. The skin is the largest organ in the body and accounts for 16% of the body weight. Hair are of two types: *terminal* which are long, black, and thick (androgenetic) are common in adult male; and *vellus* hair which are pale, thin and short (1mm, barely visible) on the trunk, arms, thighs and most of the face in females.

Skin

Examine for Colour (pale in anemia, yellow in jaundice, blue in cyanosis, dark in Addison's disease); Texture (rough, smooth, oily); Temperature (gauge with the dorsum of the hand); Moisture (moist or dry); Mobility; Turgor; and Lesions; excessively *sweating palms*; *sebaceous cyst; dermatosis* (non-inflammatory skin disease); *acanthosis* nigricans.

The ***lesions*** are *described morphologically* as erythema, macule, papule, nodule, pustule, cyst and wheal; and their patterns of distribution are described as linear, clustered, annular (ring like), arciform (in an arc), geographic, serpigenous (serpent-or worm-like).

Hair: The hair are examined for Quantity (sparse or luxuriant); Colour (see Chapter 4); Texture (soft or rough, oily);

Shape (straight or curly); Thinness or thickness; and Distribution. *Unwanted hair* in women and children (hirsutism); Temporal recession of scalp hair is normal in men but abnormal in women; Excessive loss of hair (alopecia); Localized sharp bordered patchy loss of hair and hair roots (alopecia areata); Dandruff; Lice in all hairy parts of the body (and clothes); and Premature graying.

Nails: The nails consist of nail bed, nail plate, nail root and paronychium. In health, they are pink, resilient, convex from side to side and flat in the long axis. Examine them for Pallor (anemia), Blue colour (cyanosis), Concavity (koilonychia), *Convexity* in the long axis as well as well as side to side with thickening of the nail bed (*clubbing*); inflamed nail margins (*paronychia*); and Local nail disorders (especially pitting and fungus infection).

Female Breasts

It drove home, personally, the value of early detection and intervention (Janet Napolitano on being detected to have early breast cancer).

The breasts are a pair of protruding, milk producing and secreting glands on the front of the chest. To describe the clinical findings, each breast is divided into four main quadrants, based on horizontal and vertical lines crossing at the nipple; the upper-outer **quadrant** is the largest. The fifth part of the breast is the **axillary tail**. The breasts consist of overlying skin, glandular tissue made of 15-20 lobes separated by fibrous connective tissue, surrounded all round by subcutaneous and retromammary fat; ducts and the appendages, areolae and nipples. Each lobe comprises numerous milk producing lobules. The ducts converge upon the nipple and carry milk to it for secretion. Its lymphatics drain mainly into the axillary lymph nodes, but also into the infraclavicular, supraclavicular and intrathoracic internal mammary nodes.

(1) Physical examination of the breast utilizes two techniques: inspection; and predominantly palpation, unimanual or bimanual, with the pads of the middle three, second, third and fourth, fingers carrying out light, medium and deep palpation.

(2) The breast is examined with the patient in the *multiple positions*, not to miss an early cancer.

(3) There is reasonable possibility of early diagnosis of carcinoma with the combination of *breast-self-examination and clinical breast examination* by a physician, done best approximately 5-7 days after the onset of menstruation, when the estrogen levels are low.

The clinical breast examination is offered in the following situations:

(a) *The patient comes with a symptom in the breast*—discomfort or pain; nipple discharge or a recent change in the *appearance* of the nipple or areola; a change in the symmetry of appearance o the two breasts—skin-redness, thickening or peau d'orange; change in the contour of a breast—dimpling, puckering, retraction; change in the size of one breast; a *suspicious breast lump felt by the patient*; a *lump in the axilla*. With a breast mass, search for axillary, supraclavicular and infraclavicular lymph nodes is mandatory. Conversely, searching the breasts for a primary is mandatory in the case of a mass in the mass in axialla.

(b) *Asymptomatic patient: age 40 years or over;* Family history of breast or ovarian cancer in close female relatives; *past history* of breast cancer in the patient; history of *benign breast disease* in the patient; history of a breast being exposed to *radiation* during radiation treatment of a neighboring organ.

The patient is conventionally examined first in the supine position, using finger tips; if there is a lumpish feel (an area that feels different from the surrounding breast tissue) palpate it with the *'flat of the hand'* (already described in an earlier chapter). The breasts are examined one at a time, quadrant by quadrant, in a predtermined manner. Do not forget the axillary tail of the breast. It can have a primary malignancy. The breast is examined in various patient positions, in order (a) not to mistake a benign nodule for a cancer; and (b) not to miss a cancer when it exists. Remember to compress nipple for discharge. Examine for ipsilateral axillay, infraclavicular and supraclavicular lymphadenopathy.

Unilateral or bilateral abnormal breast findings (e.g nipple discharge, uniductal or panductal; uni- or bilateral) help us to segregate breast lesions into benign (fibroadema or fibrocystic disease) and malignant in the first instance. The final diagnosis of cancer can be made only histologically, either by an open biopsy or after a mastectomy.

Male Breasts

Gynecomastia is a benign enlargement of the breast in boys and men (usually bilateral but sometimes unilateral) resulting from a proliferation of the glandular component of the breast. It is normal female breast development in an abnormal setting. It is defined clinically by the presence of a mass extending concentrically from the nipples.

(1) Many pubertal boys develop a *small* (less than 2 cm in diameter) soft *pad* of fat behind the areola. It is normal and not gynecomastia. It generally resolves within 1-2 years.

(2) In *true gyecomastia* early changes are a palpable, firm disk of ducts, fibrous tissue and lobule, all mixed up, and restricted to the area of the areola. It can resolve in 1-2 years. Later, the same disk may extend beyond the areola. The latter does not resolve.

Gynecomastia may occur in the normal puberal boys, elderly males; and in those with cirrhosis of the liver, hyperthyroidism, or history of estrogen or anti-androgen drug treatment. It may occur during testosterone therapy of delayed puberty in boys.

(3) In *cancer* of the male breast, the same disk is large (extends beyond the areola), hard, irregular shape, with distortion of the shape of the areola and nipple; axillary nodes may be enlarged; therefore, palpate for the axillary lymph nodes in every male with breast enlargement

(4) In **pseudogynecomastia**, which occurs in obese boys, the discrete central disk is absent and there is only a mass of fat, looking like a female breast. This is also called lipomastia.

Axillae

Normal: See chapter 4

The axillae are the hairy spaces between the chest wall and the right and left arms. They are examined by inspection and palpation. They emanate an odour in adults.

Inspection: Hair—Sparse (always so or recent loss) or luxuriant.

Skin—Evidence of infection (furuncle i. e. boil); lice.

Skin—Over-pigmented (deodorants or frequent depilation especially chemical depilation); acanthosis nigricans;

Palpation—*Axillary* tail of the breast; *tenderness* +/-; *lymph* nodes; *mass*; *cancer*—primary in the axillary tail of the breast or meatstases from the main breast; evidence of thrombophlebitis.

Smell: An *odour* from the axilla is normal in adults. In the case of a *stink*, a breast cancer should be considered.

Upper Limbs

Examine

- The skin and the nails.
- Muscle development; reflexes.
- Sensation.
- The hands, elbows, arms and shoulders.
- Do not forget the epitrochlear lymph nodes.
- Skeletal deformities, if any.
- Joints: range of motion and muscle strength at all joints.
- Radial and brachial pulses.

Do this, all the time comparing the two sides.

Chapter 26

Thorax and Lungs

I hereby present to the readers a new sign (Percussion) which I have discovered for detecting diseases of the chest (Joseph Leopold Auenbrugger).

The thorax is open to inspection. With the help of the anatomical surface landmarks which are real, and the virtual vertical reference lines on the surface of the thorax, we can divide the surface of the thorax into multiple zones. They tell the physician which part of the invisible lungs and mediastinal structures lies under a given zone. This is helpful to the examining physician and the operating surgeon.

The **real landmarks** are (a) Clavicles; (b) Suprasternal notch; (c) Sterno-manubrial junction with which the costal cartilage of the second rib articulates; (d) The ribs which are counted downwards from the second rib; (e) Nipples in men, in whom they are close to the mid-clavicular lines; their position in women is inconstant; (f) Xiphoid process of the sternum and costal angle; (g) Inferior angles of scapulae and (h) Spinous process of the seventh cervical vertebra.

The **virtual, vertical reference lines** are (a) Mid-sternal line; (b) Mid-clavicular line; (c) Anterior axillary line; (d) Mid-axillary line; (e) Posterior axillary line; (f) Scapular line and (g) Vertebral line.

Whereas the thoracic cage is bilaterally symmetrical, some of the intrathoracic organs are asymmetrical (a) *numberwise* e.g. the left lung has two lobes, whereas the right lung has three. and (b) *positionwise* e.g. the heart is more on the left side than the right side of the midline.

An easy way to remember the correspondence between the thoracic surface and the lobes of the lungs is as follows:

- Both the lower lobes occupy the bottom ¾ of the posterior chest fields.
- The right middle lobe is in the right axilla.
- The lingula of the left lung is in the left axilla.
- Both the upper lobes are under the anterior chest wall and top ¼ of posterior chestfields

Learn this by heart, and while auscultating, say to yourself "I am now auscultating over the...lobe". And so also with percussion.

The intercostal space between two ribs is numbered by the rib above it.

Normal: See Chapter 4 and 6.

The protocol of the examination in systems in the body is as follows:

(1) **The R.S. and the C.V.S.** are examined in the order: Inspection, Palpation, Percussion and Auscultation(**I.P.P.A.**). In the C. V. S. examination, palpation has now replaced percussion in the estimation of the heart size.

(2) The **abdomen** is examined in the order: Inspection, Auscultation, Percussion and Palpation **(I.A.P.P.)** because auscultation gives important information about the frequency of bowel sounds, and percussion and palpation of the abdomen may distort (in fact, increase) the frequency of bowel sounds.

(3)The **C.N.S.** examination has its own protocol (See C.N.S.).

General observations: Vital signs (T. P. R.); Clubbing; Cyanosis;

Edema; Frontal headache; Lymph nodes; Evidence of Cardiac failure; Type of breathing; Hands warm or cold; Patient's position in bed; Smoking; Dust or pollen exposure.

The Chest Examination

The front and lateral sides of the lungs are examined in supine position. The back of the lungs is examined with the patient sitting up. Do not auscultate the back of the lungs with the patient in either left or right lateral recumbent position (Chapter 19) because the greater ventilation in the dependent lung can lead to false asymmetry in physical signs between the two lungs (Bates).

Inspection, smell and hearing:

- Normal respiratory rate is quoted variously as from (12-18) breaths per minute to (16-25) per minute (McGee); rapid due to recent physical activity and to acute respiratory infection; slow in opioid poisoning.
- Breathing quiet or noisy.
- Visible effort of breathing.
- **Type of breathing:** Normal; shallow or deep; slow or rapid; Cheyne-Stokes; Sighing = loud, slow deep inspiration and expiration (patient is anxious and complains of not getting enough air); Deep rapid breathing of metabolic acidosis (Kussmaaul breathing).
- **Size of the chest:** Chest circumference is variable. Chest expansion is 5-13 cm at 18 diminishing to about 2.5 cm at 70.
- **Shape of the thorax:** Normal; Flat, Barrel shaped, Pigeon breast, Funnel chest, Rickety rosary and Straight back syndrome.

- Asymmetry of size, shape and movement between two sides are because of lung collapse, pleural effusion or pneumothorax; the chest moves less on the diseased lung. Asymmetry may also be secondary to spinal kypho-scoliosis.
- **Patient's posture:** A severely breathless patient may sit up in the bed; one in respiratory distress will adopt the tripod position, sitting or standing, leaning forward and supporting the upper body with hands on the knees or on another surface such as the bed.
- **Signs inspiratory obstruction:** Movement of ali nasi; Stertor (obstruction above larynx); Use of accessory muscles of inspiration (strenomastoid, scaleni, trapezius); Sucking in of intercostal spaces, suprasternal notch, supra-clavicular spaces and epigastrum (paradoxical movement of abdominal muscles); The larynx moves up and down with respiration.
- **Signs of expiratory obstruction:** Visibly prolonged expiration; Audible wheezing (their disappearance indicates worsening of the condition in severe asthma); Pursing of lips during expiration; Use of accessory muscles of expiration (abdominals and latissimus dorsi).
- **Combined severe inspiratory and expiratory distress** with choking in stridor (obstruction at larynx or distally).
- Gross lump or localized depression of the chest wall.
- Obviously visible deviation of the trachea to right or left;
- Displacement of apical cardiac impulse due to cardiomegaly, or a respiratory cause.
- **Foul smell at the bedside:** Bronchiectasis or lung abscess (Chapter 22).

- **Heard at the bedside:** Quiet breathing is inaudible at the bedside; Harsh noisy breathing; Rales (now called crackles) bubbly sounds, more commonly during inspiration); Rhonchi, (now called wheezes), whistling sounds, more commonly during expiration, due to bronchospasm); Stertor, Stridor (respiratory obstruction) (Chapter 22).

Palpation

(1) Tenderness, swelling, subcutaneous emphysema.

(2) Confirm equality of respiratory movements on two sides.

(3) Palpable rhonchi, pleural rub.

(4) Confirm the position of the trachea and cardiac apex beat by palpation.

(5) Tactile vocal fremitus (normal, increased, decreased)—compare on two sides

(6) Measure chest expansion.

Percussion: Percuss (a) gently; (b) from the expected resonant area to expected dull area; with the pleximeter finger parallel to the expected border between resonant and dull areas; (c) for an audible percussion note and the tactile vibration against the pleximeter finger.

Percuss the chest for (a) Lung borders; (b) Upper border of the liver, and its movement downwards during inspiration; (c) Equality of resonance in the mirror image areas of the chest wall on the two sides; (c) The presence of any abnormality on percussion; (e) Cardiac size (now palpation has replaced percussion for this purpose).

Percussion notes and their characterstics: (a) Flat as if percussing the thigh; (b) Dull as if percussing the liver; (c) Resonant as if percussing the healthy lung; (d) Hyperresonant as if percussing the emphesymatous lung or a pneumothorax; and (e) Tympanic as if percussing the gastric air bubble.

Auscultation

(1) Breath sounds:

(a) **Character:** Normal vesicular (faint like leaves rustling in the breeze; no gap between inspiratory and expiratory phases; expiratory sound shorter in time and feebler than inspiratory sound). Asthmatic (no gap between inspiratory and expiratory phases; expiratory phase longer than inspiratory phase); Bronchial (loud; expspiratory phase longer than inspiratory; gap between the two phases). Tracheal breathing: Like bronchial but louder.

(b) **Intensity:** Compare intensity over mirror image areas on two sides. Sometimes breath sounds may be vesicular and loud as in a child: called puerile or harsh.

(2) Foreign sounds:

(a) **Rales:** intermittent, bubbly sounds of various intensities, produced by fluid in the respiratory tract and by thickening of the alveolar walls as in fibrositis. Describe them as fine, medium or coarse.

(b) **Rhonchi:** Continuous musical sounds produced by narrowing of bronchi or by tough, vibrating strings of mucus stretching across the lumen of bronchi. Describe as low pitched or high pitched. See whether they diminish after voluntary coughing.

(c) **Pleural rub.**

(3) Vocal resonance (normal, increased or decreased).
Aegophony; Whispering pectoriloquy.

Physical signs in the respiratory system are recorded with reference to (a) Side—right or left; (b) The *intercostal space*; and (c) The *virtual vertical reference lines* (see above). This indicates which lobe of which lung is involved.

Back and Spine

With the patient's back facing you:

- Inspect the skin and the thoracic configuration.
- Inspect symmetry of the shoulders and thorax; and upper musculoskeletal development.
- Inspect and palpate scapulae and the spine, and thump with a fist gently on the spine for tenderness.
- Palpate and percuss the costovertebral angles.
- Test all movements of the spine.
- Look for tenderness anywhere.

Chapter 27

Cardiovascular and Lymphatic Systems

Sometimes, the heart sees what is invisible to the eye (H. Jackson Brown).

They are considered together because the lymphatic vessels are somewhat analogous to the caplllaries: both connect to the venous system and, through it, to the heart, and carry excess interstitial fluid, protein and locally produced metabolic waste products centripetally to the heart. The capillaries also carry blood back to the heart, which lymphatics do not do.

The physical examination is carried out and recorded in the order: inspection, palpation, percussion and auscultation (I.P.P.A.). The findings are recorded under **peripheral** (vascular and lymphatic vessels), and **central** (the precordium).

Cardiovascular System

General observations: Vital signs (T.P.R.); Weight gain due to edema; Chest pain; Dyspnoea; Anemia; Cyanosis; Hands warm or cold, Skin moist or dry; Rheumatic activity; Diabetes; Lipids; Kidney function; Smoking; Alcohol; Daily salt intake.

Peripheral Physical Signs

Arterial side:

(1) **Pallor:** Localized pallor indicates local ischemia; generalized pallor suggests anemia or shock.

(2) **Cyanosis:** It imparts blue colour to affected parts of the body. Cyanosis of the extremities, fingers, car

and nose is peripheral cyanosis. The affected parts are cold to touch. The cyanosis of lips, tongue, oral mucosa and palpebral conjunctiva is central cyanosis. The centrally cyanosed parts are normally warm to touch.

(3) **Arteries:** Radial, ulnar, brachial, carotid, femoral, popliteal, dorsalis pedis,and posterial tibial are the commonly palpated arteries. Record their presence or absence and equality or otherwise on two sides. The radials and cartotids are examined and recorded in every patient; others are examined and recorded selectively. The absence of palpable ulnar pulse is a normal variant. A systolic arterial bruit (murmur) may often be harmless. A diastolic murmur is pathological. A Systolico-diastolic arterial bruit on any artery indicate proximal, partial occlusion or stenosis of a large artery or aorta. A bruit on the liver suggests a malignancy.

(4) **Arterial pulse:** (a) Pulse rate per minute, counted for ½ minute; (b) Rhythm—regular, regularly irregular, irregularly irregular as in atrial fibrillation. Count heart rate for 1 minute, instead of pulse rate, in atrial fibrillation; (c) Volume—normal, low or high; (d) Character of arterial pulse pressure wave form -- normal, weak, bounding (water-hammer), bisferiens, alternans and bigeminal (d) Condition of the arterial wall—normal or thickened; (e) Effect of respiration on pulse rate (sinus arrhythmia) and on volume (pulsus parodoxus).

(5) **Blood pressure** is measured by palpation and auscultation. For details, see Chapter 23.

(6) The Ankle/Brachial Index measures the adequacy of foot circulation.

(7) Normally, the radial and femoral arterial pulses are palpable almost simultaneously. If the femoral pulse is significantly delayed after the radial, (Radio-Femoral delay), it indicates coarctation of the aorta.

Venous side:

The following are important:

(a) **Edema:** localized or generalized; pitting=venous; non-pitting=lymphatic; the latter may look like peau d'orngae (orange skin); (b) Distinguish between arterial and venous pulsations in the neck; (c) Measure the jugular vein pulse pressure; (d) Decipher the pattern of jugular venous pulse wave; (e) Venous varicosities in the lower limbs; (f) Evidence of chronic venous stasis and venous thrombosis, particularly in the lower limbs; (g) Evidence of obstruction in superior/inferior vena cava; (h) Evidence of obstruction of portal vein, with development of collateral circulation seen in the abdominal wall; determine the direction of blood flow if collateral veins are seen.

Special Signs: Capillary pulsations; Durozier's sign; dancing carotid and brachial arteries; tracheal tug in aneurysm of the aortic arch; venous hum.

Central (precordial) Physical Signs

(a) The heart is located in the mediastinum, immediately behind the sternum and extends beyond the left border of the sternum; (b) The right ventricle occupies most of the anterior cardiac surface. This is the position of the right ventricular heave which produces a strong forward thrust (heave) of the overlying sternum; (c) The clinical term **'base of the heart'** refers to the superior aspect of the heart at the right and the left second interspaces next to the sternum; (d) The left ventricle, behind the right ventricle and to the left, forms the left lateral border of the heart; (e) Its tapered inferior tip is termed the **cardiac apex**. This impulse is located in the left 5th intercostals space, 7-9 cm lateral to the midsternal line, at or just medial to the left midclavicular line; (f) The hypertrophied left ventricle produces strong +/-prolonged apex beat.

Location

The word **location** (of heart sounds and murmurs) is used to mean the area of the precordium where a heart sound or a murmur is heard the loudest (Point of maximal intensity; **P.M.I.**) It does not coincide with the surface marking of the concerned valve, but is downstream to it.

Inspection and Palpation of the Precordium

Inspection and palpation:

(1) Shape; Bulging; Precordial excavation, Pigeon breast.

(2) *Pulsations in an area not expected are abnormal.* They are best looked for with a tangential beam of light.

(a) The apex beat, also called the Point of Maximal Intensity (P.M.I.): describe its Location and Quality: (easily felt, difficult to locate, strength and duration; felt in another location than its normal location it is abnormal). Apex beat is not always palpable even in normal persons (normal variant). It is difficult to find it in women because of the overlying breast.

(b) Left parasternal—right ventricular heave (confirmed by palpation).

(c) Left second interspace—dilated pulmonary artery.

(d) To the right of the sternum: displaced heart or dextrocardia.

(e) Right second interspace—aneurysm of aorta.

(f) Suprasternal notch (aortic)—not necessarily abnormal.

(g) Epigastric: Normal (in thin persons)—minimally forceful, non expansile, systolic (RV inflow).

Aneurysm of aorta—expansile, post-systolic.

Right ventricular hypertrophy—transmitted, systolic in epigastrium.

Abdomen para-vertebral—aortic aneurysm, expansile and post systolic.

Pulsating liver----tricuspid regurgitation, end systolic.

(3) Parasternal retraction is seen in isolated LV volume overload due to counter clockwise twist of heart in systole.

Percussion

Percussion the heart borders: inferior border is not percussable. See if the dullness on percussion extends beyond the apex beat—consider the possibility of pericardial effusion. This is all about its usefulness in routine precordial percussion.

Palpation has largely replaced percussion in estimation of cardiac size (Bates).

Auscultation: Auscultation is the very informative part of cardiac examination. We auscultate the heart for heart sounds; extra sounds; murmurs; *and pericardial rub.*

Heart sounds: Heart sounds are discrete bursts of auditory vibrations of varying intensity (loudness), frequency (pitch), quality, and duration. The first heart sound is produced by the closure of mitral and tricuspid valves; it is heard the loudest at the apex; and it is single. The second heart sound is produced by closure of the aortic and pulmonary heart valves; and it is heard the loudest at the base and is split during inspiration (aortic component before the pulmonary component) in healthy persons. Third and fourth sounds are generally not audible. Systolic ejection clicks are high pitched and occur in early, mid- or late systole. Opening snap of the mitral valve occurs in early diastole and is a high pitched sound.

Heart sounds are characterized by: Location; Pitch; Intensity; Duration; Timing in the cardiac cycle; whether the second sound at the base is single or split physiologically; pathologically widely, fixed, or paradoxically.

Additional sounds: Pericardial rub; and sound from a mitral or aortic valve prosthesis.

Murmurs: A *murmur* is a series of vibrations of variable duration, emanating from the heart or an artery, *generally* audible with a stethoscope touching the body. It is due to turbulent blood flow in the chambers of the heart or in an artery. A grade 6 cardiac *murmur* is, however, *still audible* through the stethoscope after it is just lifted from the chest wall. Systolic cardiac murmurs may be either innocent or pathological. Diastolic cardiac *murmurs* are always pathological.

Murmurs are characterized by: Location; Pitch; Intensity (Grade I to Grade VI); Timing in the cardiac cycle; Pattern (whether crescendo or decrescendo); Radiation; Preferred position of the patient; Effect of respiration and exertion.; and Constancy from day to day. Accompanied by a palpable thrill?

Auscultate the entire precordium first with the diaphragm and then again with the bell.

Auscultate with the diaphragm in the following areas for heart sounds and murmurs:

- **Aortic area:** (a) Aortic valve second heart sound. (b) With patient supine, and then sitting and leaning forward, best for the aortic valve murmurs, especially of aortic regurgitation. Murmur of aortic regurgitation may be heard along a line from the right parasternal second space to the apex.
- **Pulmonary area:** (a) Pulmonary valve second heart sound. (b) With patient supine best for pulmonary valve murmurs.
- **Low left sternal edge:** Four intercostal spaces below the pulmonary area. With patient supine best for tricuspid valve murmurs, especially that of regurgitation.
- **Apex:** (a) First heart sound and opening snap of the mitral valve. (b) With patient supine, and then rolled over partly or fully on the left side. The turned position is best for the murmur of mitral valve stenosis.
- In the known **area of radiation of the murmur** (axilla, carotid artery and from aortic area toward and up to the apex); and
- **Inching** from apex to base or the other way round.

Below are shown the important physical signs of valvular lesions in the Heart.

Abbreviations: MA= Mitral area; AA= Aortic area; PA= Pulmonary area TA=Tricuspid area; RVH=Right ventricular hypertrophy; LVH= Left ventricular hypertrophy; MDM=Mid-diastolic murmur; EDM=Early diastolic murmur; JV=Jugular vein; RBBB= right bundle branch block.

Mitral stenosis (M.S.): (1) RVH; (2) First sound loud at apex; (3) Opening snap of mitral valve at apex; (4) MDM or presystolic, low pitched murmur at apex; accentuated in the left lateral position after exercise; no radiation (5) Thrill at the apex common.

Mitral regurgitation (M.R.): (1) LVH; (2) Pansystolic murmur at apex; radiates into left axilla; (3) EDM, a third heart sound or atrial fibrillation may be present; (4) Thrill at the apex common.

Aortic stenosis (A.S.): (1) LVH; (2) Ejection systolic murmur at AA or apex; radiates into carotids; (3) Ejection systolic click over LV; (4) Thrill at AA common.

Aortic regurgitation (A.R.): (1) LVH; (2) High pitched decrescendo EDM at AA or left 3rd interspace parasternally; radiates to the apex; best heard with patient sitting, bending forward, breath held in expiration; (3) Collapsing pulse; (4) Thrill rare.

Pulmonary stenosis (P.S.): (1) RVH; (2) Second sound widely, fixed split; (3) Systolic murmur at PA; no radiation; (4) Ejection systolic click over RV.

Tricuspid regurgitation **(T.R.):** (1) RVH; (2) Pansystolic murmur; at left, low, sternal edge; increases during inspiration; (3) JV pressure elevated, and prominent 'a' wave; (4) RBBB and atrial fibrillation frequent; (5) Pulsating liver; (6) Diagnostic accuracy very high for T.R. (Chapter 20).

Tricuspid stenosis (T.S.) (acquired): (1) Absent RVH; (2) Mid-diastolic or presystolic murmur, which accentuates during inspiration, at the lower end of the sternum; (3) Opening snap +/-; (4) Split first heart sound and single second heart sound; (5) A prominent 'a' wave in JV; (6) Liver pulsates.

Lymphatic System

Except for the placenta and the brain, every tissue that is supplied by blood vessels also contains lymphatic vessels. They carry back into circulation the interstitial fluid in excess of what is carried back by the blood capillaries. On their way back there are lymph nodes; they carry out multiple functions including being a part of the immune system. They are either superficial (subcutaneous) or deep (in thorax, abdomen and pelvis). Only the superficial lymph nodes are palpable during physical examination; The superficial nodes are arranged in groups viz. the cervical, axillary, epitrochlear, and inguinal nodes. Tonsils and thymus are other lymphatic organs.

There are three physical signs in disease of lymphatic system (1) Enlarged lymph nodes (larger than 1 cm in adults; lymphadenopathy or lymphadenitis); (2) Lymphangitis—tender, red streaks in the skin, extending to infected lymph nodes; and (3) Lymphedema=non-pitting edema. It may be pitting in the early stage.

Physical examination of the lymphatic system comprises:

- Inspection and palpation of the above mentioned areas for lymph nodes as they are normally impalpable; when palpable they are round or oval encapsulated masses. Describe their site (single site i.e localized; or multiple sites i.e. generalized); size (less than 1cm in diameter or larger); size; discrete; matted (= stuck to each other); shotty (=tiny, round, discrete like a pellet of gun-shots; consistency normal, firm, caseous = having the feel of cheese because of central necrosis as in tubercular lymph nodes; hard as in cancer); mobility; whether painful, tender.

- When palpable and larger than 1 cm; ·they need investigation for infection or primary malignancy i.e starting in the area or organ where it is palpable with no lesion in its area of drainage), or secondaries from lesion in its area of drainage, which you should search for.
- Examine for palpable lymph nodes in all lymph node areas, and for palpable spleen.
- Tender, red lines of lymphangitis.
- Non-pitting edema (of feet as in filariasis, or of arm as after radical mastectomy).
- Palpable epitrochlear, infraclavicular and supraclavicular lymph nodes are ominous because of probability of primary cancer or serious generalized infection (including AIDS), and secondary cancer (primary being in the chest or abdomen as in the case of supratrochlear nodes).

Chapter 28

Abdomen

Gastrointestinal Tract; Liver and Gall Bladder; Spleen; Kidney; Urinary Tract and Prostate

---

The abdomen is a Pandora's Box (Greek mythology).

The abdomen is a multi-system, multi-organ conglomerate (= a group or mixture of different things). The organs are the gastrointestinal (G.I.) tract, the liver, the spleen, kidneys and the urinary tract.

Many times, abdominal complaints surprisingly and unexpectedly are found to have an extra-abdominal cause.

Gastrointestinal Tract

The physical examination of the G.I. tract is carried out and recorded in the order: inspection, auscultation, percussion and palpation ***(I.A.P.P.).*** *This is because percussion and palpation may stimulate the frequency of bowel sounds (Bates).*

The front of the abdomen is divided into nine regions by two imaginary horizontal and two imaginary vertical lines. The regions are, *from right to left*, (top row) right hypochondrium, epigastrium and left hypochondrium; (middle row) right renal, umbilical and left renal; and (bottom row) right iliac or inguinal, hypogastrium and left iliac or inguinal). It helps the physician to describe the location of the examination findings e. g. tenderness or a mass, and thus narrows the diagnostic possibilities.

General observations: Vital signs (T.P.R); Anemia; Stomatits; Nutritional status; Weight loss; Edema; Food habits;

Alcohol; Tobacco in any form; Jaundice; History of blood transfusion; Mass in the abdomen; Lymph nodes; Prominent veins on the abdomen

Abdomen is examined in the sequence: Inspection, Auscultation, Percussion, Palpation.

Inspection

Mouth: "It's better to remain silent and be thought a fool than to open one's mouth and remove all doubt" (Mark Twain).

Normal: See Chapter 4. The gums may be lighter pink in people with lighter skin; and brownish in dark-skinned people; these are racial normal variants. The upper surface of the tongue has papillae with associated taste buds; the undersurface has none.

Examine for: (a) *Lips:* Colour; Pigmentation; Moisture; Cracking, Signs of vitamin deficiencies, excoriations and ulceration, especially at the angles (cheilitis andangular stomatitis) (b) *Oral mucosa (Stomatits):* Colour; Moisture; White patches;. (c) *Gums and teeth:* Unhealthy gingival mucosa; Gingivitis; Pyorrhea and recession of gums. Count the residual teeth; Alignment between upper and lower teeth; Caries; Staining due to chewing tobacco or paan (betal leaves); (d) Look at the *hard and soft palate* for signs of ill health and ulceration; (e) Tongue: Asymmetry (wasting of one half); Taste buds; Pallor, Smooth dorsal surface (glossitis); Small ulceration of the tongue margins due to malaligned upper and lower teeth (tongue biting); major tongue biting (epilepsy); (f) Palpate any mucosal ulceration or nodule (cancer and pre-cancer); (g) Look for healthy or unhealthy openings of parotid and submandibular ducts; (h) Open mouth with dry oral mucosa (mouth breathing); (i) foul breath (halitosis).

- Teeth: Number, health; missing, false, carious. Alignment between upper and lower teeth.

- Mucosa of the tongue and cheeks: moisture, colour, pigmentation, ulceration; papillae of the tongue.
- Gums: Gingivitis (inflammation of gums), ulceration, recession, pyorrhea, hypertrophy, pigmentation.
- Throat and tonsils: Evidence of acute and chronic inflammation; enlarged tonsils.

Abdomen

The patient should be lying supine on the examination couch, with arms folded across the chest, not above the head. This is because, in the latter position the abdominal wall stretches and tightens, making palpation difficult.

The physician should stand on the right side of the patient. When looking for peristalsis, he should sit or bend down so the he can view the abdomen under tangential light.

- *Shape and contour:* Flat, rounded, protruberent, scaphoid (markedly concave or hollow).
- Ask the patient to take a *deep breath and hold it.* An umbilical or incisional hernia becomes prominent. Ask him to raise the head from the table. An extra-abdominal mass becomes more prominent.
- *Generealized bulging:* Five Fs (fat, flatus, fluid, faeces, fetus). Measure circumference with a measuring tape at the level of umbilicus.
- *Localized bulge:* lump? Hernia (see below for detailed description of an abdominal lump).
- *Movements with respiration:* Bulging of abdominal wall during inspiration: normal; or paradoxical movement i. e. retraction of abdominal wall during inspiration, due to severe weakness or paralysis of both hemi-diaphragms.

- *Umbilicus:* Normal, deep or everted; and its position.
- Look for Pigmentation; Branding marks; Striae; Spider nevi; Scars of past surgery.
- *Visible veins:* Direction of blood flow? portal vein obstruction? inferior vena cava obstruction?
- *Visible pulsations:* not necessarily abnormal; may be seen in thin normal persons.
- Visible peristalsis and its direction.
- Visible coils of intestines.

Auscultation: Auscultate all nine regions of the abdomen for bowel sounds (see above for reason). Apply the diaphragm gently for auscultating the abdomen. It is used for listening to bowel sounds (normally 5-34/minute); bruits; and friction rub over the liver and the spleen.

Some healthy persons have an epigastric systolic bruit which is considered normal. On the other hand, a systolic-cum-diastolic bruit strongly suggests arterial stenosis or a partial occlusion of the aorta or a large artery. Listen for hyper-peristalsis. Silent abdomen: you have to auscultate for 5 minutes before diagnosing silent abdomen. A bruit over the liver suggests hepatic carcinoma. A friction rub heard over the liver or the spleen suggests inflammation of the peritoneum over the underlying organ.

Percussion: For details see Chapter 18.

Percuss all the regions for: (a) Resonance of the normal abdomen; (b) Presence or absence of hepatic dullness; (c) Vertical span of hepatic dulness (from upper border to lower border of the liver); normally, it is 4-6 cm in the midsternal line and 6-12 cm in the midclavicular line; (d) Horse-shoe shaped and shifting dullness; (e) Fluid thrill; (f) Whether an Organ or a Lump is resonant or dull; and (g) Hepatic hydatid thrill in appropriate circumstances.

Palpation: It may be light, medium or deep. Palpate for (a) General sense of resistance; (b) Tenderness on palpation; (c) Rebound tenderness; (d) Palpable viscera (hollow viscera, liver, spleen, kidneys); (e) Lump (describe in detail as shown below); (f) Dipping; (g) Gastric splashing.

Description of an abdominal lump: (1) Whether intra-abdominal, extra-abdominal or in the abdominal wall; (2) Whether abdominal or pelvic; (3) Position with reference to the nine abdominal regions; (4) Size in centimeters, (5) Shape; (6) Tenderness; (7) Surface: whether smooth, irregular or nodular; (8) Borders: well defined: sharp, well defined and rounded or ill defined; (9) Consistency: soft, firm or hard.. Is the consistency uniform or varying? (10) Is it pulsatile (transmitted pulsation e.g. liver or expansile pulsation e.g. normal aorta or its aneurysm); (10) Movement with respiration e.g. liver or spleen; (12) Can it be moved about with your palpating hand? (13) Ballotment; (14) Resonant or dull on percussion.

Digital rectal examinations of anus, rectum and prostate

- Sim's position in men and women: The patient in left lateral, recumbent position (Chapter 19) rolled toward a prone position, buttocks close to the examination table near you. Top leg bent fully at the hip and knee; the bottom leg flexed slightly.
- Preferably Lithotomy position (Chapter 19) in women because it also allows genital examination.

In the male

- Wear gloves. Look at the anal margin and perianal skin (hairless, coarse and more pigmented) for any abnormality. During and after pushing a finger into the anal canal and rectum, feel for tone of sphincters, tenderness, induration, irregularities, nodules in the mucosa, and a mass. On withdrawal of the finger, look at it for stool, if any, its colour and for blood. See below for prostate.

In the female, the cervix, a retroverted uterus and a possible pelvic or adnexal mass can be felt.

Liver and Gall Bladder

The liver is inspected, percussed, palpated and auscultated.

Inspection for pulsating liver (tricuspid regurgitation).

Pecussion: Percuss gently from resonance to dullness. Percuss the upper border and the lower border in the midclavicular line.

Measure the vertical span of the liver in cm. Percuss for tenderness on the right lateral side,

Thump gently with a fist on the right lobe of the liver to elicit tenderness.

Palpation: Palpate lightly first and heavily later if necessary.

Place the left hand on the right lower posterior aspect; palpate in front with the right hand.

Palpate from the umbilical upward towards to right costal margin. The lower edge of right lobe of the liver is not palpable in healthy persons except on taking a deep breath; when palpable, the liver edge is normally soft, sharp, regular and smooth. Feel for consistency, tenderness, irregularity.

It descends as much as 3 cm with deep breath.

Look for tenderness.

The left lobe is palpable below the costal margin up to 4-6 cm.

Auscultate the liver for a bruit or a rub; if bruit present, it suggests malignancy.

Examine for a palpable gall bladder under the liver edge at the border of the right rectus abdominis. A healthy gall bladder is not palpable. A palpable, tender gall bladder indicates cholecystitis. If gall bladder is palpable in a jaundiced patient, it is unlikely to be due to gallstones; it suggests pancreatic malignancy. (Courvoisier's law).

Look for jaundice and ascites.

Spleen

The spleen is located deep in the left hypochondrium. A normal spleen is not palpable in 95% of normal persons. It has to enlarge to twice its size to become palpable below the costal margin. It is palpable rarely i.e. in 5% of healthy adults (Bates). Therefore, a *palpable spleen is almost always abnormal.* The spleen enlarges in the *inferior anteromedial* direction, sometimes as far as the right iliac fossa.

Palpation: Start palpating in the right iliac fossa (so that you do not miss a giant spleen) and move gently towards the left costal margin. Ask the patient to take a deep breath. Dr. Rosenberg recommends in Stanford Medicine 25 as follows "Do not dip your fingers. *Let the spleen palpate your fingers, not the other way around. There is no gold; so, do not dig*. Some enlarged spleens are very fragile and are liable to be injured".

When palpable, it has a sharp edge and a notch.

If the spleen is not palpable with the patient in supine position, make him turn into right lateral recumbent position (Chapter 19) and palpate again. If doubt persists, get ultrasonography done. *It is safer and more decisive than palpation and percussion.*

Percussion: Percussion suggests but does not confirm a spleen (Bates). Its sensitivity and specificity are moderate.

Auscultate for a rub (inflammation of the overlying peritoneum).

Kidneys and Urinary Tract

Thorough symptom evaluation (see System Symptom Review, Chapter 13) and routine urine examination form the diagnostic backbone of disorders of the Kidneys and Urinary tract. There are few physical signs to elicit in this system. They are 'Local' and 'Systemic'.

Local physical signs:

(1) **Abdominal** examination for tenderness in the lumbar regions; a mass in the lumbar region consistent with a renal mass; hypogastric tenderness; inappropriately full bladder; arterial bruit in the upper abdomen consistent with renal artery stenosis.

(2) **Urethral** discharge; tenderness or a lesion in the male external genital organ (penis) or female external genital organs (vulva); perineal tenderness.

(3) **Prostate:** During the rectal examination (see above) palpate the lateral lobes of the prostate for: shape, size (normal or enlarged), consistency, lump tenderness and the mobility of the prostate. Anterior and median lobes are inaccessible during rectal examination.

Systemic physical signs:

(1) Hypertension and its consequences.

(2) Clinical evidence of contracted plasma volume (dehydration, low blood pressure, postural hypotension), or expanded plasma volume (edema or congestive failure).

(3) Clinical evidence of renal failure.

Asymptomatic patient: Routine urine examination in an apparently healthy person may show an abnormality (protein, red blood cells, pus cells) which needs to be investigated. This situation may arise in a person who comes for a routine annual check up or for a life insurance medical examination.

Investigations: Appropriate investigations (imaging) may be urgent (within minutes to hours) or leisurely (within hours to days). They are generally definitive diagnostically.

Chapter 29

Groins, External Genitals and Lower Limbs

Don't lift my words without permission. It might lead to a hernia (Jarod Kintz).

Groins

General observations: Hernia: Having to strain at coughing, passing urine or stool. Lymph nodes.

Inspection

Area above the inguinal ligament

- Hernia.

Area below the inguinal ligament

- Hernia.
- Enlarged lymph nodes.

Palpation

Area below the inguinal ligament: Hernia or Lymph nodes (horizontal and vertical chains); femoral artery aneurysm; thrombosed femoral vein.

Female Genital Organs

General observations: Sexual maturity; normal sexual intercourse; pregnancy; gravidity and parity; post menopausal—osteoporosis, fracture (hip, spine, jaw); sexual practices and sexual violence.

According to The American College of Obstetricians and Gynecologists (ACOG), the pelvic examination includes three elements:

(1) *Inspection* of the Labia; Clitoris; Uurethral meatus; Vaginal introitus; and Perianal region (**external examination**). Examine them for Inflammation; Ulceration; Discharge; Swelling or Nodules; and evidence of Sexual trauma. Finally look for any evidence of Lesions of Sexually Transmitted Diseases (S.T.D.).

(2) **Speculum examination** of the vagina and cervix; and

(3) **Bimanual examination** of the uterus, cervix, and adnexa. (2+3 constitute the **internal examination**). When indicated, a rectovaginal examination also should be performed.

Such examination is offered (1) when the *patient has symptoms* in the concerned parts; and (2) to well-women on annual visits. The latter is a matter of debate, especially about the age at which the visits should start, the frequency of the visits and the extent and details of examination. The purpose of the annual examination is annual health assessment, promoting prevention practices, recognizing risk factors for disease, identifying medical problems, and **establishing the clinician–patient relationship**. (See N.E.J.M. 5-11-2015 for merits).

With exceptions, *women prefer a lady doctor for a gynec examination on their own selves*. This is so even in an advanced country such as the U.S.A. where most doctors allow a female patient to specify the gender of the examining doctor. A chaperone nearby is a must; and people who are not directly concerned should be requested to leave the examination room.

Male External Genitals

General obversations: Complaint of small penis; Erectile dysfunction; Sexual habits; History of S.T.D.; Urethral discharge; Local trauma.

Examine the patient standing naked and facing you

- Pubic hair, including lice.
- Penis, urethral meatus including urethral discharge and its nature.
- Roll back the prepuce and look carefully for any lesion and old scars.
- Scrotum and its contents: testes (note their size), epidydimes, spermatic cords, especially the vast deference. One testis (more commonly the left) hangs lower than the other; it is a normal variant.
- Testis is a very sensitive organ; it hurts even on minimum pressure. So be very gentle while examining it.
- Look for a hydrocele.
- Look for tenderness and swelling anywhere.
- Elicit cremasteric reflex.

Always keep eyes alert for symmetry.

Lower Limbs

The following are examined by inspection, palpation and certain other manoevres in the lower limbs with the patient lying supine:

Skin: Looks healthy? Discoloration; Dry or Moist; Warm or Cold; Smooth or Rough; Scratch marks; Excoriations; Ulcer;

Loss of hair; Toe nails normal? Evidence of infection; Cutaneous lesions of leprosy.

Lymph nodes: inguinal, mainly vertical group.

Hernia.

Circulation: Pitting or non-pitting edema; Varicose veins; Venous thrombosis. Palpate arterial pulses (femoral, popliteal, dorslia pedis, posterior tibial); Ankle/brachial index; Gangrene-dry/moist.

Nervous system: Muscles—Bulk; Tone; Strength; Wasting; Sensation---Pain (monofilament test); Vibration; Thickened lateral peroneal nerve (leprosy); Reflexes. knee, ankle and plantar reflexes; Foot drop; Bones---Tenderness, Evidence of old fracture.

Joints: Hips, knees, ankle, big toe----deformity, swelling, tenderness, range of motion; gouty tophi.

Feet: (The curse of diabetes)

- Dry skin; Scratch marks; Excoriations; Ulcer; Loss of hair; Wasting of small muscles; Impaired popliteal and ankle arterial pulses; Diminished sensation especially pain and vibration sense; Sensory ataxia; Loss of ankle jerks; Deformities; Charcot foot; Gangrene.

There are many other non-routine tests possible in patients with special problems.

Chapter 30

Physical Signs in Diabetes Mellitus

Managing diabetes is not science; it is an art based on science (Anonymous).

There is hardly any tissue or organ in the body that **diabetes mellitus** does not affect. Symptoms are too numerous to be included in this chapter. Therefore, this chapter lists for you **abnormal physical signs in diabetes which, by definition, can be verified clinically**, and are either suggestive of diabetes or a complications of diabetes. They will be listed in 'head to toe' sequence as far as possible. In this small book, it is possible only to enumerate them but not describe or discuss them. Symptoms are not given, nor are laboratory or imaging tests. The remaining neurological signs are listed in a separate cluster at the end.

Infections are one of the commonest complications

Skin: Boils; Carbuncles; Dry skin; Loss of hair especially in the feet; Patchy areas on the trunk which *perspire after meals*; Scratch marks; Excoriation marks; Diabetic dermopathy; Either *dark skin* or *acanthosis nigricans* in many different sites; *Xanthomatosis; Hirsutism* in women; *Thickening of the skin* of the back of the neck and upper back.

Face and associated organs:

- Facial wrinkle.
- Dry mouth; oral infections; delayed healing after dental surgery; gum disease.

Eye: Eyelid and conjunctival infection; impaired vision, chronic or acute; arcus senilus; cataract; dry eye syndrome; diplopia due to an oculomotor nerve palsy; recurrent corneal erosion syndrome; chalazion.

External ear: External auditory canal infection; malignat otitis externa.

Neck:

- Dark skin or acanthosis nigricans; narrowed carotid arteries with a bruit.

Axilla:

- Dark skin or *acanthosis nigricans; lymphadenopathy* due to diabetic mastopathy; hydradenitis supporativa; *Addison's disease; contact dermatitis.*

Hands:

- *Painful* hands; *tenosynovitis; stiff* hand syndrome; *Dupuytren's* contracture; *Carpal* tunnel syndrome.

Thorax and lungs:

- Obtructive sleep apnea.

Heart and circulation:

- *Tachycardia* (early manifestation of parasympathetic autonomic neuropathy); signs of heart failure (elevated jugular venous pressure; orthopnea; cardiomegaly); *ischemia* due to poor circulation e. g. feet; *orthostatic* hypotension; postprandial *hypotension.*

Weight:

- Weight gain; weight loss.

Abdomen:

- Elevated waist circumference (*central obesity*); deep umbilicus.

Female external genitals:

- Scratch marks; excoriations; dark skin or acanthosis nigricans; vulvitis; vaginitis; yeast infection.

Male external genitals:

- Scratch marks; *excoiations; yeast* infection; *balanitis* or *balanoprosthitis*; phimosis; dark skin or *acanthosis* nigricans.
- *Erectile* dysfunction; *priapism; Pyronie's* disease.

Feet: See Chapter 29

Other neurological signs:

- *Bell's* palsy; *T.I.A.; stroke;* mono- or poly-peripheral *neuropathies* of several distributions and producing a variety of clinical pictures; *diabetic coma.*

Chapter 31

Central Nervous System

Activity of the nervous system improves the capacity for activity, just as exercising a muscle makes it stronger (Dr. Ralph Gerard).

General observations: Trauma; Infection; Features of Parkinsonism, Chorea, Myasthenia, Adenoma sebaceous. Muscle disease; T.I.A.; Atial fibrillation; Diabetes; Abnormal posture: Hemiplegic, Paraplegic. Long-standing history of boxing, Contact sports; Alcoholism; Therapeutic drugs. In the elderly; No regular mental activity in elderly; Generalized atherosclerotic disease.

Out of the physical examination protocols of subspecialties of internal medicine, that of the C.N.S. is the most rigorous and the most 'technique dependent' (see Chapter 7). It must be personally taught by a teacher. In addition, CDs holding videos of C.N.S. examination are now available, and they bear repeated viewing. The written description of the technique can supplement bedside teaching/videos but cannot replace them.

The protocol for nervous system examination is: (1) Mental status (Higher functions); (2) Cranial nerves; (3) Motor system; (4) Sensory system; (5) Reflexes and (6) **Gait**; (7) Romberg's sign; and (8) Others.

Gait is the most important neurologic sign because normal gait requires that the four areas of the nervous system function in an integrated way. They are (1) *Motor system for muscular strength*; (2) *Cerebellar system* for rhythmic movement and steady posture; (3) *Vestibular system* for balance and for coordinating eye, head and body movements; and (4) *Sensory system* for position sense.

Clinical pearls (Harrison's book):

(1) Neurologic examination may be normal in a patient with a serious neurologic disease e.g. seizures or T.I.A.

(2) Uncommon presentations of common diseases are more likely than a disease with rare etiology e.g. Alzheimer's disease is commoner than a prion disease.

(3) Diagnose a treatable disease such as a nervous system infection, an acute stroke or spinal cord compression rather than an esoteric disease.

Minimum (or screening) neurologic examination

These tests are meant to be carried out by physicians other than neurologists in a patient who has no neurologic complaints, in order to adequately screen for abnormalities.

Mental status: Ease of communication; orientation in time and space; recall and insight into recent and past events.

Cranial nerves: Optic fundi; visual fields of both eyes together; pupillary size and reactions; extra-ocular movements; and facial movements

Motor System: Muscle strength and atrophy in limbs; and extremity tone.

Sensory system: Light touch and warm or cold temperature in each distal extremity; and simultaneous, double sensory light touch with examiner touching patient's one or both hands, with patient's eyes closed.

Reflexes: Biceps, patellar and Achilles reflexes.

Coordination: Observe the patient at rest and during

spontaneous movements. Rapid alternating movements of hands and feet; finger-nose test.

Gait: Observe the patient while walking in his usual style; on heels and on toes; and walking heel-to-toe (Tandem walk).

After practice, this entire test is said to be completed in 3-5 minutes.

Full Neurologic Examination

Mental status, also called Higher functions:

(1) Appearance; motor behaviour; spontaneous vocalization; dress, grooming and personal hygiene.

(2) Level of consciousness.

(3) Speech and language: normal, dysarthric or aphasic.

(4) Memory: recent and past.

(5) Orientation in time and space.

(6) Common general knowledge.

(7) Abstract thinking.

(8) Look for illusions, hallucinations, delusions and delirium which are fairly common conditions; look for their cause. Depression and dementia more serious mental disorders

These make up the mental status for which tests are described.

Cognition is all the mental processes that, put together, underlie our use of five senses, orientation, attention, memory, information, vocabulary, calculations, abstract thinking, and constructional ability, which are collectively responsible for learning, acquisition of knowledge and building experience.

Cranial Nerves (CN)

1st CN: Olfactory— Rule out common cold. Test the ability to *recognize and identify* the presence of an odour. Use a common, non-pungent substance such as coffee, cloves, soap, vanilla or asafetida; but not *ammonia or camphor.*

2nd CN: Optic— Visual acuity; field of vision first with both eyes simultaneously, then one eye at a time; colour vision and optic fundi.

3rd CN (Occulomotor), 4th CN (Trochlear) and 6th CN (Abducens): These are tested together.

- Look for ptosis; proptosis; diplopia; nysagmus; conjugate deviation; and squint (paralytic or non-paralytic).
- Ocular movements: One eye and both eyes: Command movements; Follow movements; and conjugate movements. Nystagmus- its direction is the direction of the fast component. A few nystagmoid movements at the extreme of lateral gaze is a normal variant.

2nd and 3rd CN: Pupils: Size; shape; position; equality of size and reaction to light and to accomodation. Tiny difference between the size of the two pupils cannot be identified clinically.

5th CN (Trigeminal): Motor division: Muscles of mastication: masseters, temporals and pterygoids for movement (opening and closing mouth and moving the jaw from side to side—the jaw deviates to the paralyzed side); strength (clenching jaws and biting); muscle wasting; and jaw jerk.

Sensory division: (a) Corneal reflex; (b) Sensation on face. The trigeminal nerve picks up irritant odours; so do not use them in testing 1st CN.

7th CN (Facial): Motor function: Test facial muscles for expression, position and wasting; facial movements (closing and opening the eyes and smiling)., and facial deformity therefrom.

Sensory function: Sense of taste on the anterior 2/3rds of the tongue on one side at a time: sweet (sugar), salty (table salt), sour (sour lime), bitter (quinine); and umami (ripe tomatoes, dry cured ham, certain cheeses); the last group of substances imparts not only a taste but a meaty flavor to the food due to their content of monosodium glutamate.

8th CN Auditory nerve: Cochlear division: (1) Examine the external auditory canal ear for inflammation and excess of wax; ear drum for perforation. (2) Test for acuity of hearing (whispered voice test; ticking watch test); (2) Test air and bone conduction (Rinne's test); and lateralization (Weber's test).

Vestibular division—(1) Stance (the way of standing) and gait; (2) Positional nystagmus; (3) Refer the patient to the E. N. T. department for caloric test.

9th CN (Glossopharyngeal), 10th CN (Vagus) and 11th CN (Cranial accessory): are tested together; they cannot be tested individually:

Motor function: Position of the uvula and the arches of the soft palate. Movements of palate, uvula, pharynx, larynx; hoarseness of voice; stridor. Abnormal speech (dysarthria i.e. poor articulation although speech formation and contents are normal).

Sensory function: Taste sensation on the posterior 1/3rds of the tongue, supplied by the ninth CN, is not tested routinely.

Combined motor and sensory functions: gag reflex tests both components. Its absence in the absence of any other abnormality is a normal variant.

11th CN (Spinal accessory) nerve: Sternomastoid muscle, upper part of the trapezoid muscle—atrophy and strength.

12th CN (Hypoglossal): Tongue—Symmetry; atrophy and fasciculations (with tongue in the floor of the mouth); deviates to the paralyzed side (on attempted protrusion of the tongue).

Motor System

(1) Position of the body at rest and during movement.

(2) Strength refers to the amount of force a muscle can produce with a single maximal effort. Tested isotonically and isometrically. Describe the result as normal or weak. Test successively in various muscle groups at all joints. Compare the two sides. Describe the degree and distribution of weakness. In certain cases, test the strength of individual muscles. Are voluntary movements slow or clumsy?

(3) Tone is the slight, residual tension which a normal muscle with an in tact nerve supply retains even after the it relaxes. It is tested by passive movement of a muscle by the examiner. It may be normal, increased or diminished. The increased tone may be either clasp-knife type (in pyramidal lesion) or lead pipe/ cogwheel type (in extra-pyramidal lesion). Diminished tone is found in lower motor neurone lesion and at the onset of a pyramidal lesion. Describe the distribution of the abnormal tone.

(4) Nutrition: Do the muscles look appropriate in size for the age, gender, occupation, exercise taken/games played, or sedentary habits? Do they appear wasted? Is the wasting selective or generalized? Are they enlarged (hypertrophied) and strong (true hypertrophy), or hypertrophied but weak (pseudohypertropy)? What is the distribution of hypertrophy or pseudohypertrophy?

(5) Involuntary movements? (a) Tremor: type and distribution; coarse or fine? frequency; speed; exaggerated at rest/ during movement; effect of sleep; does it satisfy the criteria of essential tremor? (b) Chorea. (d) Athetosis. (e) Myoclonus. (f) Tics. (g) Asterixis.

What is the patient's age? Is there evidence of anxiety/tension, therapeutic drug consumption, habitual alcohol consumption, evidence of hepatic cirrhosis or psychiatric disease?

(6) Coordination: Posture; gait (normal; hemiplegic; paraplegic; high steppage; parkinonian; and ataxic); finger-nose test; heel-knee test; and rapid alternating movements; these are cerebellar signs.

(7) Signs of parkinsonism; meningeal signs (meningitis).

(8) Contractions or deformities.

Sensory System

Abnormality of sensation: Diminished sensation (numbness, hypoalgesia); absent sensation (anaesthesia); increased sensation (hyperesthesia and hyperalgesia); and dysesthesia (feeling otherwise than the normal feeling of touch).

The types of sensation tested are:

(1) Superficial: Light touch, pain, temperature.
(2) Deep: Pain (muscles, testicles), vibration and joint sense (position, movement).
(3) Cortical: Tactile localization, tactile discrimination, tactile lateralization, stereognosis.

If sensory deficit is present, what is its pattern? To what neuronal innervation does it correspond? Distribution of sensory roots? Individual nerve(s)? Glove and stocking? Hemi? Upper horizontal level in the trunk—spinal cord lesion; crossed hemi-anaesthesia.

Reflexes

The reflexes are of two types: Tendon reflexes and cutaneous reflexes.

Tendon reflexes: When you briskly tap the tendon of a partially stretched muscle, the muscle suddenly contracts. This is called a tendon reflex. It is a spinal reflex and may involve a single spinal segment (monosynaptic) or more than one segments (polysynaptic). Each reflex involves specific spinal segments and therefore tendon reflexes are valuable in localizing the spinal cord lesions. Normally, they are bilaterally symmetrical. Pathologically, they may be exaggerated (upper motor neurone lesions) or diminished in intensity (lower motor neurone lesions; and in certain other types of clinical conditions e. g. hypothyroidism). In some diseases, they are not elicitable—they are said to be absent. They can be graded from hyperactive to absent on an ordinal (ranking) scale. Reinforcement has to be used to be convinced about their real absence. Their generalized absence may sometimes be a normal variant.

The commonly elicited tendon reflexes are: biceps reflex; triceps reflex; supinator reflex; knee reflex (knee jerk)and ankle reflex (ankle jerk). They are 'technique dependent' for correct interpretation. So, learn the proper way of doing them from your teacher.

Cutaneous reflexes: (1) Abdominal reflexes: These are elicited by stroking the abdominal skin from lateral to medial aspect with a blunt object in all four quadrants. The response is a deviation of the umbilicus toward the area stimulated. (2)The plantar reflex is highly technique dependent.

Others: Trophic changes; skull and spine; tetany; nerve root irritation (S L R test).

Chapter 32

Diagnosis and Record Keeping

Bedside manners are no substitute for the right diagnosis (Andrew Weil).

Admission summary: After completing the history and physical examination, make a brief yet complete summary. This would include important points from your clinical *examination* and from patient's concerns (see Empathy in Chapter 12).

Provisional diagnosis and differential diagnosis: These diagnoses are made on the basis of your clinical examination of the patient.

- If the patient's illness can be explained by one single disease, then, it is straight-forward **provisional** diagnosis, to be confirmed or refuted by tests and the course of the illness. Enter it in the patient record file, along with the reasons for making the diagnosis.
- If you think that the illness needs more than pathological process to explain the patient's all problems, write down the list of possibilities that you think of, in the order of likelihood; this is **differential** diagnosis. Especially the elderly often have multiple pathologies. Write down the arguments for and against each diagnosis.

Analyze the contribution of each factor to the total illness. Such factors are (1) **environmental** i.e. geographical, cultural and socioeconomic; (2) **psychological** i.e. patient's mental make up and attitude; and (3) **pathological** i.e. the disease process itself. (d) One may add the genetics to this list now.

Proposed investigation: They fall into three groups:

- **Routine:** They are to be done on every patient to assess his general state of health. They are hemogram, E. S. R., urinalysis, fasting blood glucose, creatinine; TSH and vitamin D, the last two, if the patient can afford them, as these conditions are common and treatable.
- An X'ray of the chest and an E.C.G. may now be considered as routine tests.
- **Specific:** They are done on the basis of data available so far e.g. liver function tests, ultrasonography, bone densitometry, cardiac stress test and so on. They help to pinpoint the diagnosis. They should be done with the knowledge of what you are going to do with the result.
- **Research:** These are done to study a specific problem in depth. They should be ordered only after knowing what you will do with the results. With the availability of multitest autoanalyzers, doing multiple biochemical tests has become easy.
- The addition of **nuclear medicine tests** has expanded the vista of chemical and imaging tests very much.

Treatment plan: See Chapter 2 on medical record. All the cautions given there apply also to the prescription, only more so. Oral orders can be risky and therefore tabooed. The prescription must always be written on a letterhead, dated and signed.

Progress notes: These should be written regularly, (though the frequency may vary), and in addition if and when the patient is seen by you out of his routine turn. Specialists invited to give an opinion must give it in writing. The notes comprise any change in patient's symptoms and physical signs, results of investigations done and patient's response to treatment. Any alteration in the treatment must be entered in the record.

Final diagnosis: This may turn out to be the same as admission diagnosis or may be different. It must be unambiguously entered in the patient record. Additional problems or complications may have arisen during the course of illness. They and their management must be recoded. The final total diagnosis will include (a) anatomical diagnosis, (b) physiological or functional diagnosis, (c) pathological diagnosis and (d) etiological diagnosis. Write clearly the solved problems and those that are alive at the time of discharge.

Advice about further treatment and frequency of follow up: This is important and may turn out to have a medicolegal angle at a future date.

Discharge summary: It is customary and courteous to forward a summary of the important events during the patient's hospital stay to the referring physician. It also gives you a colleague to look after the patient on day-to-day basis. This makes it safer for the patient and time saving for you.

Also read Chapter 2.

Tables

Table 1: Hemoptysis vs Hematemesis

Hemoptysis	Hematemesis
Preceded by cough.	Preceded by epigastric discomfort or pain.
Blood is coughed.	Blood is vomited.
Blood is bright red and frothy.	Blood is clotted and dark.
Alkaline in reaction.	Acid in reaction.
History of smoking or tuberculosis.	History suggestive of peptic ulcer, cirrhosis, alcoholism; ingestion of aspirin or a glucocorticoid.
Physical signs of lung disease.	Physical signs of stomach or liver disease.

Table 2: Pyramidal vs Extrapyramidal Lesion

Pyramidal lesion	Extrapyramidal lesion
Weakness (partial or complete) present.	No true weakness present.
Clasp-knife increase in tone (spasticity) present in anti-gravity muscles.	Lead-pipe or cog-wheel rigidity affecting flexors and extensors in limbs.
No involuntary movements.	Involuntary movements may be present.
Rapidity and refinement of movement lost out of proportion to weakness.	Movement hindered by rigidity and loss of initiative.
Emotional movements present and may even be exaggerated.	Emotional and associated movements depressed.
Tendon reflexes brisk.	Tendon reflexes normal.
Plantar reflex extensor.	Plantar reflex flexor.

Table 3: Upper and lower motor neurone paralysis

Upper motor neurone paralysis	Lower motor neurone paralysis
Paralysis of movements.	Paralysis of muscles.
Voluntary but not emotional movements lost in affected muscles.	All movements lost in affected muscles.
Fine movements lost out of proportion to weakness.	All types of movement impaired or lost.
No or minimal wasting.	Gross wasting may be present.
Spasticity except during stage of shock.	Always flaccid.
Tendon reflexes brisk.	Tendon reflexes absent.
Plantar reflex extensor.	Plantar reflex.
No reaction of degeneration.	Reaction of degeneration present at appropriate stage.

Table 4: Pulsations in the neck

Arterial	**Venous**
Movement is sharp and localized.	Movement is soft, diffuse and undulant.
Can be felt.	Cannot be felt.
Single pulsation.	Double pulsation at normal heart rate and rhythm.
Top level of the pulsation constant.	Top level changes with phases of respiration, abdominal pressure and posture.
Does not cease on light compression at the root of neck.	Pulsation cease on compressing the jugular vein at the root of the neck.

Appendix 1
Characters of a Liver Lump

(1) Liver is situated in the right hyopchondrium and epigastrium.
(2) Left lobe of normal liver may be palpable in the epigastrium.
(3) Moves freely on breathing.
(4) The lower edge of right lobe may be palpable during deep inspiration; in that case, it is sharp and regular. Its surface, if palpable, is soft and smooth
(5) Fingers cannot be insinuated between the lump and the costal margin.
(6) Dull on percussion; and dullness continuous with that of normal liver dullness.
(7) Tenderness on palpating liver edge and on thumping gently on the right lobe.

Appendix 2
Characters of a Splenic Lump

(1) Spleen is situated deep in the left hypochondrium.
(2) A normal spleen is generally not palpable (95%). Rarely, the tip of a normal spleen with a long pedicle may be just palpable under the left costal margin (5%).
(3) A palpable spleen is almost always abnormal.
(4) The spleen enlarges downwards and rightwards. It may reach the right iliac fossa.
(5) Moves freely with breathing.
(6) When felt, anterior border is sharp and has a notch.
(7) Fingers can be insinuated between the posterior border and the spinal muscles.
(8) The fingers cannot be insinuated between the lump and the costal margin. Therefore, upper border cannot be defined.

(9) Dull on percussion anteriorly.

(10) Not ballottable.

Appendix 3

Characters of a Kidney Lump

(1) The kidneys are situated in the right and lumbar regions.

(2) They move freely on breathing..

(3) Borders are rounded.

(4) Lower pole of normal right kidney is palpable on inspiration. Bimanual palpation produces sickening pain.

(5) Fingers can be insinuated between the lump and the costal margin. Therefore, the upper border can be defined.

(6) Fingers cannot be insinuated between the lump and the spinal muscles. Therefore, posterior border cannot be defined.

(7) Resonant on percussion anteriorly.

(8) Ballottable on bimanual palpation.

Appendix 4

Physical Signs of Ascites

(1) Generalized bulging of the abdomen, more so in the flanks.

(2) Umbilicus may be flat or everted.

(3) Normal or increased sense of resistance on palpation.

(4) Viscera palpable on dipping.

(5) Horse-shoe shaped dullness.

(6) Shifting dullness.

(7) Fluid thrill in tense ascites.

(8) A very small amount peritoneal fluid cannot be made out on physical examination. Ulltrasonography is required to demonstrate it.

(9) Physical signs of the cause e. g. cirrhosis of the liver may be present.

List of Sources of Information Used

(1) Physical Diagnosis by Golwalla and Vakil. 14th Edition.

(2) History Taking and Clinical Diagnosis by D.D. Vora, 2nd Edition.

(3) Barbara Bates' Guide to Physical Examination and History Taking, 11th Edition.

(4) Mosby's Guide to Physical Examination, 7th Edition.

(5) Hutchison's Clinical Methods 23rd Edition.

(6) Walker, Hall and Hurst's Clinical Methods 3rd Edition.

(7) Evidence Based Physical Diagnosis, by Steven McGee, 3rd Edition.

(8) French's Index of Differential Diagnosis, 15th Edition.

(9) Williams, Textbook of Endocrinology, 12 Ed. Chapter 3.

(10) Calm Sutra, The Art of Relaxation by Nadkarni Dilip, 1st Edition, Pub.: The Times of India, Mumbai.

(11) Harrison's Principles of Internal Medicine. 9th Edition.

(12) History Taking and Physical Examination by Bhandarkar S.D,. 2nd Edition

(13) Websites.